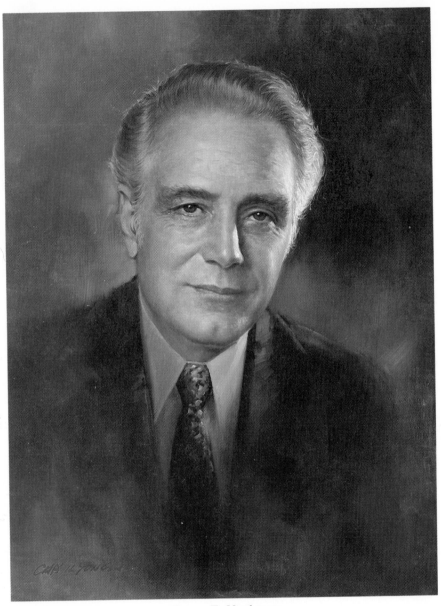

George E. Vandeman

IT IS WRITTEN CLASSICS

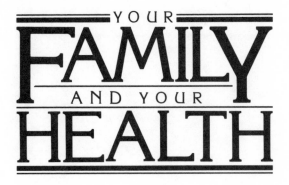

YOUR
FAMILY
AND YOUR
HEALTH

GEORGE E. VANDEMAN

Pacific Press Publishing Association
Boise, Idaho
Montemorelos, Nuevo Leon, Mexico
Oshawa, Ontario, Canada

Edited by Ken McFarland
Cover design by Tim Larson
Portrait of George Vandeman by Ilyong Cha
Type set in 10/12 Century Schoolbook

First Printing 1986: 7500

ISBN 0-8163-0643-5

Contents

In Appreciation

This volume is the first of four which present the heart of my ministry in permanent form. Other minds than mine have combined to bring "It Is Written" the success it has enjoyed. To the Lord Jesus Christ I eagerly give credit. I also owe no small amount of appreciation to Nellie, my loving and faithful companion in a lifelong commitment of service for others; to three fine sons, George, Ronald, and Robert; and a lovely daughter, Connie. Each one of them has helped to keep me humble, human, and happy.

And I owe much to my office family as well—a skilled and faithful team of workers who live and breathe the ministry to which we're all committed. Outstanding among these has been Marjorie Lewis Lloyd, always an able writer and researcher, who for thirty years assisted in the production of the "It Is Written" program. To all of these I owe very much indeed. But to the Unseen One—my Friend—goes the eternal credit for the vastly more important dimension that will make these books live in the hearts of all who read them.

Before You Turn the Page

Throughout Pastor Vandeman's thirty years of television ministry, two extremely popular subjects will be particularly remembered as classics. First, his warm, understanding, and penetrating insights on home and marriage. You will not find it difficult to identify with him as he relives the secrets of success in these very personal areas of life.

And simply reading the chapter titles in the second section will kindle, the publishers believe, a genuine desire to discover the way to radiant health. Understanding preventive medicine, seeking a new lifestyle in harmony with our Creator's plan, can do wonders in healing body, mind, and soul.

One other observation will be helpful to the reader before turning this page. Please remember that these chapters are in reality scripts of telecasts that have been released over the years on topics of lasting interest. These chapters/scripts are arranged in as natural a sequence as possible. However, since they were first scripts and not book chapters and since they present the great truths of Scripture, there may be some repetition which, though minimal, should be understood.

Pastor Vandeman believes that essential truths of Scripture need to be released to the public by way of television, more than once or twice, from fresh and helpful but different perspectives. Actually, this repetition or review is intended for the public's good, and it is hoped the same benefit can accrue to the reader as well.

A Word From Paul Harvey—

One of the books which made a lasting impact on my own perspective is *Planet in Rebellion* by my treasured friend, George Vandeman.

Perhaps not since the songs of David has profound truth been reduced to its essence with such shirt-sleeve eloquence. And he has done it again—and again.

And now again. This time in four pertinent volumes.

George Vandeman's books speak as he speaks—and when he speaks of home, marriage, and health—he practices every precept which he recommends.

After twenty-five books in a dozen languages, this harmonious quartet is an appropriate literary crescendo in the career of a one-of-a-kind disciple.

Read and reread in digestible doses at bedtime if you can. I do.

Paul Harvey

Happiness Wall to Wall

It's an exciting moment when one man and one woman are launched together into the swift-moving waters of matrimony—with happiness just downstream. But what do you do if, out in the rapids, the raft comes apart? Do you attempt to tie the pieces together? Do you look for a branch that might hang out over the current, close enough to grasp? Do you call for help?

Bill, in San Diego, looks up from his noonday sandwich and startles his friend with the question, "Say, you have a happy home. What's your secret?"

Sandy, in Detroit, speaks softly into the telephone. "I know, Mom. I never thought it could happen to us."

Bob, in Wichita, steps into a quiet waiting room. A few minutes later in the private office, he says, "I never thought I'd ever see a marriage counselor. But maybe you know some secret that I don't. God knows I've tried."

Carol, in New York, sits across from her pastor in his study. "I don't know what has gone wrong. We both expected happiness. But it has been a straight road into a living hell."

Kent, in Chicago, looks his father straight in the eye. "Dad, do you think there is any way of picking up the pieces now—after all this? I guess we read the road signs wrong, or something. Our marriage just didn't take."

The raft has come apart. And disillusioned husbands and wives from Maine to California are trying to tie the pieces together. They are looking for some sturdy branch which they

7

can grasp in a final attempt to hold the raft steady. They are calling for help, each in his own way, but with the same common desperation.

And then, one spring morning, a little irritated by the clear blue sky and the singing of the birds, Bill in San Diego, Sandy in Detroit, Bob in Wichita, Carol in New York, and Kent in Chicago, step into elevators—grim and determined and beaten—push the button for their floor, and walk into the office of their attorney. They are filing for divorce.

They don't want divorce. They don't believe in divorce. They have tried to postpone this day. But home has become something even worse than an open marital breakup.

Each of them is about to become another statistic. These five abandoned marriages will be included in 450,000 divorces granted this year. As statistics, ten disillusioned marriage partners will join the fifteen million other Americans who are divorced. Their children? They will join the ranks of four million boys and girls who, as the aftermath of divorce, must face the future with half, or less than half, the parents they deserve.

But Bill and Sandy and Bob and Carol and Kent are more than statistics. They are human beings. The one nagging thought in their minds is that they have failed in life's greatest adventure. Their pride and their self-confidence are undermined.

Sandy and Carol find themselves disorganized, moody, unable to concentrate, worried about the children but with no one to share their concern. They are bitter, overwhelmed, and lonely.

Bill and Bob and Kent are haunted by the fact that their own children don't really belong to them anymore—and never will.

The children cry themselves to sleep at night because they still love both parents—and feel guilty because this is so.

Yet Bill and Sandy and Bob and Carol and Kent, with their mates, five or ten or fifteen years ago, stood in happy anticipation before the altar—like countless couples from many generations—and repeated after the minister, "Till death do us part." They clasped hands as they heard the words, "What therefore God hath joined together, let not man put asunder."

Never were promises more eagerly made. Their every dream included the word *forever*. What has happened? Why have their promises become only statistics? What is the secret of lasting marriage? What is it that keeps untainted, unmarred, unshattered, the inexpressible joy of the wedding day?

Is marriage nothing more than candlelight and romance that soon burns out? How does it work in a five-room house with four walls, three children, a restricted budget, and a custom-made problem or two? Can there still be happiness—wall to wall?

The truth is that locked within the marriage contract lie either the potent seeds of devastating emotional difficulties, or the strong foundations for enduring success. Which will it be? Will marriage be a ceremony—or a creation? Will it be a duel—or a duet? Will the raft carry you safely to happiness? Or will it come apart?

Reminds one, doesn't it, of the winsome prayer of the Brittany fishermen? "Keep us, O God! The sea is so big, and our boats are so little!"

Is marriage always what the partners expect it to be? Does it obediently follow their blueprint?

A lovely young wife, after four years of marriage, was discussing needed marital adjustments with her pastor. Charming in her feminine chatter, she turned back into the fairyland of her courtship dreams. She had been wedded in a beautiful church service to a fine young man. She looked forward to never-ending enchantment, travel, affection without end, clothes fit for a princess, and barrels of money. Yes, and endless energy to enjoy all these things—like a bubbling artesian well.

Now she seemed to say, "Why didn't you tell me that there would be a shift of scenery?" She sensed now that she would have to accept the realities of homemaking. She needed to adjust to babies, dishes, bills, and hard work without compromise.

No marriage is a feature-length romance of ecstasy. Even the best marriages are the product of pull and stress, strain and concern. Successful relationships are forged in the crucibles of daily tasks and daily challenges.

Yet what man would be courageous enough when he proposed marriage to ask, "Would you be willing to work eighty hours a week for me for nothing? Would you cart home from the market and prepare something like 500,000 pounds of food? Would you wash a mountain of dirty dishes as large as a sizable ski jump—just for love? Will you wash and iron the clothes on a line forty-seven miles long with two extra miles of specialty items added for each baby? Will you climb to the top of the Washington Monument for me 12,000 times—just for love?"

No. Marriage is not an endless honeymoon. It is an endless sharing of the tasks and responsibilities of making a home. The newness will wear off. The glamour of courtship will not always continue. But does the fabric of spontaneous companionship have to wear as thin as it does?

In early marriage the husband extends his hand and helps his wife alight from the car as if she were a Cinderella on her way to a ball. But now, if she delays a moment, he walks ahead and calls back, "Come on, honey. We don't have all day!"

Does it have to be that way?

In courtship days he often admires the softness of her hands. He is captivated by her date-fresh hairdo. True, her hands, in time, may show a little dishpan red. Her hairdo may suffer an occasional tussle with the wind. But does the husband, looking forward to a little beauty and romance, have to come home from work only to have her meet him at the door with curlers in her hair, in a frayed housecoat, slippers that don't match, and a lifeless, unscrubbed complexion? Is it really surprising that he blurts out, "What have you been doing all day?" and goes seeking better scenery?

Is such a letdown inevitable? Do marriages really have to deteriorate from the very beginning? Must reality always bring disillusionment?

One young couple had dated under the usual social conditions. But they decided to test their love in a different setting. Every night for a week he came to her home, where they cooked dinner and washed the dishes together. Then they sat in the living room and talked. No radio. No TV. No record player. They simply talked together all evening. He then said good night and walked out. They wanted to be certain, before spending a lifetime together, that they could stand each other under such realistic conditions without being bored.

You see, happiness is not a state of continuous laughter, perpetual excitement and hilarity. It is not found in continual flitting from one fun spot to another. Happiness is the preparing of a meal. Happiness is watching little children grow from infancy to adulthood. It is cooking and freezing, spading the garden, washing the car, walking in the woods, shopping for the family, eating homemade bread, watching a blazing sunset.

Marriages do not have to come apart in midstream. But they will if you are not agreed on your destination. They will if the knots are not securely tied. They will if you underestimate the pull of the current. They will if you come to the rapids unprepared.

Marriage is life's greatest adventure. But it is also the most frightening voyage you can take.

You see, when you marry, you do far more than take to yourself a wife or a husband, and the obligations of marriage. You take into your hands, as a sacred trust, a bit of human destiny. The man or woman you marry is more than a body to be clothed and fed. There is a soul as well. When you face the Judge of all the earth, a time that is repeatedly and reverently described in Scripture, you stand absolutely alone before your God. But here is a matter in which you face eternal responsibility for all given to you by marriage or by birth.

It becomes mighty important, doesn't it? Worth working at. Worth building it right, beginning it right. Worth a solid foundation.

Said the psalmist, "Except the Lord build the house, they labor in vain that build it." Psalm 127:1.

How important are the foundations of a marriage? Burgess and Cotrell, pioneer researchers in the field, discovered that vows said in a religious marriage service, with the approval of both sets of parents, were most lasting. Those married by a justice of the peace were more unhappy than happy. When the husband stopped going to church before he was eleven years of age, the couple was one tenth as happy as the average. If husband and wife continued attending church until they were nineteen and attended two thirds of the time after marriage, they were 50 percent happier than the average couple.

This is just a statistical way of saying what Martin Luther discovered. After his marriage to the nun across the way, he spoke of the miracle of Jesus at the wedding feast when He turned the water into wine. Luther commented that if Jesus is not in your marriage, life is tasteless and without zest. But when Jesus comes into your home He always changes the water into wine. His presence transforms the ordinary and common routine into experiences of zest and sparkle. He takes away the drudgery. He takes away the coldness of duty and puts every-day happiness in its place.

Evidently it is possible to build a marriage so satisfying that heaven will seem to us neither far away nor strange—because our own hearthside has known the touch of heaven here and now.

But the possibilities against such a success in marriage are tremendous. There are so many places to get off course, so many potential areas of misunderstanding, so many situations that will not yield to common sense alone, so many circumstances the marriage manual does not fit, that the wonder is that any marriage ever succeeds. If it does succeed, not alone on the surface but in its unseen everyday relationships, it is because a sincere willingness to learn is combined with the miracle of the presence of Him who created both marriage and its personnel.

Marriage, I say, is a frightening adventure. It is a linking of destinies that we would scarcely risk were it not for the pull of the heart. Imagine! Two people who have never lived together, who know little about each other, suddenly undertake to live together the rest of their lives, from this day forward!

Good fortune, sorrow, failure and disgrace, sickness and health—all will be shared. And more than that, by their commitment they lay themselves open to a whole new range of dialogue and hurts and problems never before possible.

The more sensitive they are to happiness, the deeper will be the wounds. The higher the expectations, the keener will be the disappointments. The more unselfish the devotion, the more crushing the betrayal.

There will be conflict in marriage. It cannot be otherwise. For the personal intimacy that is inherent in all the everyday relationships of marriage is inseparable from a degree of conflict. Intimacy creates a certain amount of tension. In a strange paradox it creates the wounds it heals. Why? Because in marriage each partner exposes himself to the most critical scrutiny of the other. And that other has probably entered into marriage with exaggerated expectations. Reality is honest. But it is also frightening. Two distinct personalities here attempt to fuse as one. And marriage is only the beginning. To be fully known, and yet be fully loved—that is the goal.

Marriage, you see, makes each partner peculiarly vulnerable to the other. For it exposes every weakness, every difference of opinion. It exposes every failure of one to meet the expectations of the other. It opens up limitless possibilities for hurt.

When two people have joined hands in matrimony, there is no longer any room for pretense. They must abandon all masks and poses, all games. The continuous intimacy of married life will expose them all for what they are. Simplicity and sincerity are vital. Yet how rare are those virtues today! Happy is the man or woman who brings them to his marriage.

Dwight Hervey Small has said it so well: "Modern society trains us to be subtle and sophisticated, indirect and devious, clever. We live by exaggeration and affectation. We become experts at impression, masters at pretense. . . . We express emotions we do not feel. . . . We prefer the world of make-believe."— *Design for Christian Marriage,* page 59.

There is no place for pretense and parade in marriage. No place for window dressing. Only authenticity will pass the test. But you can bring to your marriage that priceless gift of genuine sincerity if you will. Success in marriage is not easy. But thank God it is possible!

Remember Bill—and Sandy—and Bob—and Carol—and Kent?

Could it be that portraits of these five problem homes could spotlight your need or mine? Are they a composite picture of marriage in distress? And if you find yourself identifying with one of them, is it not because human nature, wherever it is found, displays a likeness to itself?

Bill, in San Diego, doesn't really know what is wrong with his marriage when he asks his lunchtime friend for advice. He only knows that communication in his home is hopelessly blocked. He really blames his wife. But he is a husband who won't talk. His father was a man of few words. And he is the same. Why should his wife need reassurance of his love? He works his head off for her, doesn't he?

And now, she won't talk either. If both partners had realized that the communication system is the heart of a marriage, if some simple principles had been understood and practiced, could not this rift have been avoided? It makes one think of the words of Hosea 4:6: "My people are destroyed for lack of knowledge."

Sandy, in Detroit, would tell you a different story. She was an only child, brought up in a rather strict home. She felt her freedom restricted and seized upon an early marriage as a form of protest. At first she tried to live up to most of the principles she had been taught. Her husband admired her for it, and it looked as if their marriage might succeed. Then he began bringing home some of those stimulating, bluntly suggestive magazines and paperbacks from the newsstand. She wouldn't read them. She hid them. Then she read just one. And that was the beginning.

It was not long before the moral fiber of their marriage began to weaken. Yet, compared to what they were reading, their own activities seemed above reproach. The decay was almost imperceptible at first. But finally there was this other couple—and the wife-swapping episode that ended in divorce. Sandy would tell you it didn't need to happen.

Bob, in Wichita, thinks the trouble is in his marriage. He still doesn't realize that the trouble is in himself. He simply has not learned the basic principles that would enable him to get along with people—people anywhere, on the job, in social contacts, in any human relationship. He has moved from one job to another, never really understanding why. His wife was patient, really. They separated several times for a few weeks, but always tried it again because of the children. Finally they just stopped trying. A second marriage for Bob won't stand a chance unless he learns that the trouble with marriage is trouble with the personnel.

Carol, in New York, has experienced perhaps the most dramatic tragedy of the five. Actually, she and her husband came from almost identical backgrounds. Both came from small towns. Both had good homes. Both encountered the claims of Christ in their teen-age years. She decided for her Lord. He did not. She was counseled to reconsider the marriage. She was troubled by the words of the apostle: "Be ye not unequally yoked together with unbelievers." 2 Corinthians 6:14. But her case was different. She thought his religious background would hold him steady—even if he didn't live his convictions. Now, however, she describes their marriage as a straight road into a living hell. She can't explain it. She can only reluctantly tell it. At first their paths began to diverge only slightly. Then they moved to the city, and her husband's love for the sensational began to create a problem. He was curious about hypnotism— curious enough to want to probe just a little. Then he began to experiment with drugs—just to see what the magazines were talking about. He urged Carol to join him in his new adventures. That, of course, she could not do. Then finally came that psychedelic weekend. Marital disaster. A straight road into a living hell. And she really should have known.

Kent, in Chicago, is the man who has everything—promising job, suburban home, interesting social life, enviable bank account, a charming wife and three lovely children. That is, he did have a wife and three lovely children—until the divorce. He may find another wife to grace his home and share his social life and his bank account. But his children aren't really his anymore. And they can never be replaced.

He is the man who has everything—except an active faith in God. He is not really an unbeliever. He believes. But he wants to keep his faith boxed in so that it can't touch his work life, his social contacts, or even his home. Why should his kids have religion fed to them with a spoon? When they are old enough to make a choice, they will make a choice. His wife didn't really need to make such an issue of it. But now she has the children. The house is strangely quiet. And what went wrong with his marriage? Why didn't it take? Why wasn't it stable enough to stand a little gust of wind?

Can homes like these be saved? Can the raft be steadied and tied together before the killer rapids are reached? Can the vulnerabilities of marriage be better understood, blocks in communication removed, dangers spotlighted, personalities protected, rifts avoided, minds kept strong by facing problems honestly?

I think so. That's why you hold these pages in your hands!

Formula for Two

Happy marriage is not a glamorous package that the partners discover in the huge pile of wedding gifts. It is not something made and stored in heaven ready to be handed out to any two applicants. Rather, it is a do-it-yourself project. It has been suggested that it is like one of those kits which comes knocked down for putting together. It will take some gluing, some sanding of rough spots. Hammering a bit. Filing down the scratches. Planing, carving, bending, varnishing—and then backing off to take a look. Dusting and waxing and polishing until at last you recognize it as a dream fulfilled.

What is it that makes a house a home? What is it that transforms a collection of people into a happy family? What is it that makes a home a father's kingdom where the wife is queen, every daughter a princess, every son an heir—and where Christ reigns over all? Evidently the family tie is the closest, the most tender and sacred on earth. Listen!

> Love is not passion, love is not pride;
> Love is a journeying side by side.
> Not of the breezes, nor of the gale—
> Love is the steady set of the sail.
>
> Deeper than ecstasy, sweeter than light,
> Born in the sunshine, born in the night,
> Flaming in victory, strongest in loss,
> Love is a sacrament made for a cross.

17

I think right here you want me to share with you the Scripture formula for true love. It is not only a *formula for two,* but a formula for getting along with people anywhere. For in every relationship in life it's people that make the problem. Listen to 1 Corinthians 13:4-7, reading from the New English Bible:

"Love is patient; love is kind and envies no one. Love is never boastful, nor conceited, nor rude; never selfish, not quick to take offense. Love keeps no score of wrongs; does not gloat over other men's sins, but delights in the truth. There is nothing love cannot face; there is no limit to its faith, its hope, and its endurance."

There you have it! God's *formula for two.* Read it again and again. Evidently we are here dealing with a dimension in human relationships that has been little understood. For here is emphasized so precisely the value of the individual—the other individual. So often it has been overlooked. And as a result the partner's sense of security has been threatened.

I am not talking about a bank account. I am talking about security in the other's affections. A sense of security and a feeling of worth are as important to a man or a woman as life and health. Nothing can so quickly encourage happiness in marriage as to build in your mate a sense of security in your affection, the feeling of being valued and loved and needed. Without such a foundation happiness will have a very short life.

Check yourself by the divine formula—if you dare. I promise you, the revelation may be disturbing. At least, I found it so. Are you patient? Are you kind? Are you boastful and conceited, sometimes rude? Are you selfish and sensitive, quick to take offense? And tell me, do you keep a score of wrongs, slights, and injustices that come your way? Are you quick to watch out for your rights, careful to see that they are recognized by others?

Bruce Barton tells a little-known story from the experience of Abraham Lincoln. In the early months of the Civil War, Lincoln and a member of his cabinet went to call on General McClellan. Official etiquette prescribes that the President shall not call upon a private citizen. But the times were too tense for protocol. Lincoln needed firsthand information, and McClellan was the only man in Washington who could give it.

The General was not at home, and the two men waited in his

parlor for an hour. Finally they heard him at the door and supposed that he would speak to them immediately. But without a word he hurried upstairs. They waited another thirty minutes. Finally Lincoln asked one of the servants to remind the General that they were still waiting. After a few moments the servant returned and told them, with obvious embarrassment, that McClellan had said he was too tired to see the President. In fact, he had already undressed and gone to bed.

When the two men were outside, the cabinet member exploded in anger. Should not Lincoln instantly oust McClellan from command? But the President laid his hand on the other man's shoulder. "Don't take it so hard," he said. "I'll hold McClellan's horse, if he will only bring us victories."

Why was Lincoln willing to accept this insult to his dignity? There was a great purpose in his heart to win the war and to free a race. That was his passion. His pride, his position, his dignity, his rights took second place.

That's how the formula works in public life. That's how it works in the home. "Love seeketh not her own." The destiny of the home, the future of two souls, the happiness of our mate—these come first. Our own rights, the respect due us—these come second. Strangely enough, happiness can more easily find us when we are standing second in line.

I have discovered, too often the hard way, that the secret of lasting marriage is made up of little things—little unselfish acts, little words, little courtesies, little attentions. Why is it that we have kind words for others through the day, but when we cross the threshold of our own homes there is a tendency to let down? Why—when we love our own the best?

> We have careful thoughts for the stranger,
> Sweet smiles for the sometime guest,
> But oft for our own, the bitter tone,
> Though we love our own the best.
>   —Margaret Sangster.

The threshold of home can be a lift instead of a letdown. We need not leave tact and human kindness on the office desk. You love your family deeply. But do they know it? Do we ever find ourselves taking too much for granted?

Christianity in the home includes appreciation and kindness, culture and simple courtesy, as well as uprightness of character. Bluntness, painful frankness, the brand of honesty that prides itself on always saying what it thinks, no matter how unkind— these are not virtues, but faults. They do not belong in the home. In fact, they do not belong in any relationship.

The four walls of home were meant to enclose happiness, not to shut it out. Home should be more than a temporary shelter for wounded sensitivities and broken hearts. And it can be. When Christ is in the home, it will be a place where we give our own the best, where the simple attentions and courtesies of courtship come as naturally as the day they were born.

A choice story that my wife Nellie discovered in her reading and which I have told around the world is that of a couple about to celebrate their golden wedding anniversary. (And incidentally, did you know that, even with the eroding elements of this twentieth century, one fifth of our marriages last more than fifty years?) In this instance a local newspaper sent out a reporter for an interview, and only the husband was at home.

"What is your recipe for a long, happy marriage?" the reporter asked.

"Well, I'll tell you, young fellow," the old gentleman said slowly. "I was an orphan, and I always had to work pretty hard for my board and keep. I never even looked at a girl until I was grown. Sarah was the first one I ever kept company with. When she maneuvered me into proposing, I was scared stiff. But after the wedding her pa took me aside and handed me a little package. 'Here is all you really need to know,' he said. And this is what was in the package."

He reached for a large gold watch in his pocket, opened it, and handed it to the reporter. There across the face of the watch, where he could see it a dozen times a day, were written these words, *"Say something nice to Sarah."*

Too simple to work, you say? But it did. Remember that happiness is purchased by small, inexpensive tokens. Thoughts of appreciation pay. Criticism does not. Understanding, tender affection, freely expressed—these build a happy relationship.

But sometimes kindness and appreciation are pushed aside and forgotten. Sometimes, I have painfully discovered, there has to be some mending done, some verbal repairing, some changing of heart, some assuming of personal blame. Every marital raft fit to face the gale will have to have the ropes tied a little tighter now and then before risking the rapids.

High on the list of happy marriages that I have known about is that of Bob and Helen. Dr. Charles Shedd recalls the details.

Bob was a pusher, and she was retiring. He was the life of a party; she stayed in the shadows. Yet they seemed perfectly mated. You would see them holding hands and exchanging a sly smile as if they were reading some silent message between them.

One night they gave a dinner party. Several times Bob went to the kitchen and offered to help. Finally she let him pour the water. And then, when all was ready, he served her first! I don't know what book of etiquette he had been reading. But she sat there beaming, as if it were supposed to be that way.

The whole dinner was a thing of beauty. Several times in the conversation he asked her opinion on some subject—and even listened while she expressed it.

After dinner a guest took Bob aside and asked him the secret of his happy marriage.

"I tell you," he said, "it hasn't always been this way. The first couple of years of our marriage were pretty rough, until we were ready to call it quits. Then one day we decided to make a list of all the things we didn't like about each other. The lists were pretty long, but Helen gave me hers and I gave her mine. It was pretty rough reading. Some of the things we had never said out loud or shared in any way.

"Then we did what sounds like a foolish thing. We went out to the backyard to the ash can and burned those lists, watched them go up in smoke, while we put our arms around each other for the first time in months. Then we went back into the house, and we each made a list of all the good things we could dig up about each other. This took a little time. It was hard, because we were pretty down on our marriage. But we kept at it.

"Then we did another thing that might look silly to you. Come on back to the bedroom and I'll show you." He led his friend to the neat, attractive bedroom. And there at the focal point on the wall, in two maple frames, were two scratchy lists.

"If we have any secret, it is this," Bob confided. He told how he had memorized his list while driving to work, how he kept repeating it every day. And he said, "Now I think she is the most wonderful person in the world. And I guess she feels the same about me. That's all."

That's all? But it goes to the heart of a great marriage—this canceling out the bad and building up the good. Theirs was homemade heaven! With two scratchy lists on the wall!

Remember what Paul says? "Love keeps no score of wrongs." Take them out to the ash can—literally. Burn them up!

Friend, your relationship may need some mending. If it does, remember that the strong threads of kindness and appreciation are the most lasting material you can use.

Every home needs mending. Every home has misunderstandings. Every home has disagreements. But the longer I live and the more people I meet, the more I realize that the most delicate care must be used in settling these conflicts. For differences of opinion, in the loaded, dangerous atmosphere of criticism and blame, are highly explosive.

Here is good counsel for your home and mine. Never quarrel at breakfast. Many a husband has torn out of the driveway, spinning gravel on his way to a collision, after a breakfast-table quarrel. And many a wife has spent her day in regret. Now follow through. Never quarrel when he comes home from work. A husband can stand almost anything at work if he has a happy home. Never let him come home to a nagging wife. And then, never quarrel after the lights are out. It spoils the day.

In fact, my counsel would be simply, Never quarrel! There are no good quarrels. Let the steam off some other way. Quarrels never clear the air—they only poison it. Quarrels only scar. Current books to the contrary, a fight is a fight, whether the weapons used are fists or adjectives. Word wounds are often worse than those made by clubs.

Have you read "The First Settler's Story" recently? That time-worn tale is one of pathos, but it contains a lot of wise counsel for married hearts. You remember the young settler came home tired after a long day's work. For some reason, without his wife's knowing it, the cows had escaped. And he blamed her for it. "You had nothing else to do!" he said. "You could at least have watched the cows!"

Immediately he regretted his bitter words. But the damage was done. He felt led to beg her forgiveness that night, but his pride stood in the way. The next morning he was in a hurry and left reconciliation for another time.

Late in the afternoon he saw a storm coming up and headed for home. The cabin was empty. But there on the table was a note. "The cows have gone again," it said. "I'm sorry. I tried to keep them in. Please have kind words for me when you come home. I have gone to find the cows."

His wife? Out in that storm? He hurried after her, caring nothing now about the cows. She had not realized the severity of the storm that now broke in all its fury. While lightning tore across the sky, ripping it into deafening crashes of thunder that released a blinding hail, he searched frantically for his dear one. All night he combed the hills and valleys. Then with the morning sun he returned to the cabin, only to find her limp body lying not far from where he had killed her with his tongue. It was too late—*too late for words!*

> If I had known in the morning
> How wearily all the day
>   The words unkind
>   Would trouble my mind
> I said when you went away,
>
> I had been more careful, darling,
>   Nor given you needless pain;
> But we vex our own
> With look and tone
>   We might never take back again.
>
> For though in the quiet evening
> You may give me the kiss of peace,
>   Yet it might be
>   That never for me
> The pain of the heart should cease.

How many go forth in the morning
　That never come home at night,
And hearts have broken
For harsh words spoken
　That sorrow can ne'er set right. . . .

"Oh, lips with the curve impatient,
　And brow with that look of scorn,
'Twere a cruel fate
Were the night too late
　To undo the work of the morn."
　　　　　　　　　—Margaret Sangster.

In any home, I say, there will be differences of opinion that need to be discussed. It is a good rule never to go to sleep at night until misunderstandings have been cleared up, if there have been any. Paul says, "Never go to bed angry—don't give the devil that sort of foothold." Ephesians 4:26, 27, Phillips.

I believe you will regret any deviation from this plan. Differences are best approached in the quiet, uncharged atmosphere of tenderness and understanding, with forgiveness freely granted. For misunderstandings, if not cleared up promptly, become set in the mind as attitudes and can eventually ruin a marriage.

And now I want to ask you a question. You love your wife. You love your husband. But have you ever thought of him, or her, as your best friend? Stop just here for a moment and think it through. Your best friend. Basically, husband and wife are friends. Wouldn't this idea relax many a strained relationship?

Friends. Don't friends do things together? Don't friends share things together? Are you letting your marriage become only an assumed responsibility, rather than a spontaneous friendship? Someone has said that love is friendship set to music. Is it that way with you? Or are you trying to keep the love when the friendship has long been lost? Are you drinking from the brazen cups of duty while you could be drinking from the golden chalices of friendship?

Do things together. And it doesn't stop with husband and

wife. Every child that enters the home needs attention. He needs *two* dedicated parents. He needs their time. He needs the sacrifice of selfish plans. Happy families play together, work together, explore life together, build a boat together—even if it leaks. Just ask my boys and my daughter Connie about the boat that leaked. Go camping together. It doesn't matter so much what you do. But do it together. Memory tells me I should have done it more.

And another secret. When couples, and families, learn to pray together, they will have discovered an important factor in preventing marital difficulties. Family prayer was once an established institution. When it declined, up went home problems and divorce. The number of people who go on week after week, month after month, year after year, without family devotions, is simply appalling—many of them professed Christians.

What about prayer in *your* home? God said through Jeremiah, "My people have forgotten me days without number." Jeremiah 2:32. Makes one think, doesn't it?

In one home where a Christian mother had passed away, the little girl told a stranger in awed and frightened tones, "We haven't had prayer in our house since Mother died, and *nothing has happened yet!*"

What a poor, limited conception of what prayer really means! Are our children being taught that prayer is merely a fire escape? No, nothing had happened in that home. Nothing but slow, imperceptible decay.

God isn't going to strike us dead. He loves us too much for that. There probably won't be any serious calamity aside from spiritual disintegration. And thus gradually we lose out just when we think we are strongest.

Worship in the home, making the home Christ-centered, can be a most happy experience in the lives of our children. They need not be made to feel that prayer time is an unwelcome duty or a burden.

A word just here. The devotional program of one home may not be best for another. The schedule of family devotions will need to be tailored to the needs of your home. This is what I mean. The ideal, it would seem, would be to gather the family together for prayers both morning and evening. But suppose that you have tried it. It worked fine in the morning. But when you attempted it after the evening meal, the children complained, the phone rang constantly, and everybody had to wait. Tableclearing, dishes, and homework were all delayed. Everybody went to bed tense and cross. But you had had your family devotions!

That, for your home, may not be the best plan. Then you might try continuing with the family group together for morning worship. But at bedtime let each parent spend time individually with each child—talking over any problems, praying together. Let each child look forward to this time with Father and with Mother that is completely his own. In my own home we followed the first plan as our two older boys were growing up. Now, with our younger son and our daughter, we find the second plan happier. There is a right way, a best way, for your home. Find it—and then follow it consistently.

No amount of family devotion, of course, can take the place of your own time alone with God. But even here there is a right way—a way that will help, not prejudice, the lives that you touch. In one home the father rose early each morning for meditation and prayer alone in his den. His small daughter followed him one morning, but was told to "get out of here." She asked her mother what daddy was doing. And mother said, "He's trying to learn to love the people downtown."

Love the people downtown? And lose one's own? Fortunately that father saw his mistake, and soon it was not unusual for one of the children to join him in his morning prayer.

Is it possible to overestimate the saving influence of a Christian home? Children may wander for a while during the disturbing upheaval of adolescence. But the memory of consistent, honest dedication in the home will never be erased. God said through Isaiah, "I will contend with him that contendeth with thee, and I will save thy children." Isaiah 49:25. What a promise! And you can trust His word.

Marriage Isn't Easy

In the early days of the South a rather strange ceremony was contrived by plantation owners for slaves who desired to be married. The couple would be asked to join hands and jump over a broomstick three times. Then the plantation owner would say, "I pronounce you man and wife until death or distance do you part."

Eyebrows lift today at the thought of being married by jumping a broomstick. But I ask you, What might history say of a generation who *dissolved* marriages by rapping a gavel? Are we doing any better? Is divorce the solution? Is it an easy back door out of an unpleasant situation?

It is a sacred moment when two people who were strangers to each other are drawn together by an irresistible attraction so that they cannot from that moment be divided by time or space.

When a man sees in one woman that dream of purity and sweetness that has ever haunted his soul, or when in one man a woman finds the love and satisfaction that she has been unconsciously seeking, they can know that they have found the basis for lasting happiness.

It was to protect and prolong that sacred moment that those memorable words were spoken by Him who was the Creator, "What therefore God hath joined together, let not man put asunder." Matthew 19:6.

Countless radiant couples from many generations have echoed these words as they have repeated after the minister, "Till death do us part."

Now there are promises to keep. Will it be easy to keep them in a world where morality is treated as nothing more than an academic issue to be tossed to the experts? Will it be easy to keep them in a society whose moral fabric is tearing at the seams? Will it be easy to keep them in the days when happiness has become an uneasy peace that intermittently retreats behind the truce lines? Will it be easy to keep them in a materialistic circle that confuses happiness with possessions?

No. In a world like this, marriage isn't easy!

Unfortunately, this delightful arrangement given by God has in too many cases been so cheapened and abused that it has little resemblance to what God intended it to be. Holy wedlock has too often been transformed into unholy deadlock.

Many marriage partners—and their number is legion—are caught in a desperate struggle to save their marriage. Some are frankly confused, not knowing why or how their hopes have been so bitterly blasted. Others are distressingly aware that some personal failure is responsible for their difficulty.

As a result, divorce has assumed fantastic proportions. Someone has said, "Let's call marriage a belt that we can buckle and unbuckle." In other words, if you don't like it, just unhook!

Marriage has become a cloak, blessed and sanctioned by society, to be sure, but to be cast off at will. One young socialite flitted from one mate to another so often that a society columnist suggested the need for a wash-and-wear wedding gown. And one young man boasted before his wedding, "If it doesn't work I will have saved enough on my income tax to get a divorce next year."

God never intended that sacred relationship to be either assumed or discharged so lightly. Yet Dr. Karl Menninger, the famous Kansas psychiatrist, predicts that shortly every family in North America will be touched by divorce somewhere.

Aldous Huxley, in *Brave New World,* carries it to a shocking extreme. He wrote that if the rate of divorce continued to accelerate, "In a few years, no doubt, marriage licenses will be sold like dog licenses, good for a period of twelve months, with no law against changing dogs or keeping more than one animal at a time."

It may be all right for a spaniel, friend. But not for men and women made in the image of God.

Loose marriages, easy divorces, and broken homes are constantly yielding a harvest of bitter tears and broken hearts. Or worse still—festering wounds, deep-seated resentments, bitterness, and hatred that are actually poisoning the springs of life and inviting disease and even death.

Is there an answer to the world's marital dilemma? To whom may one turn?

Some seek the answers of popular psychology, and some have been helped. But psychology without Christ has its limitations. I have walked the floor through the night with men who were in desperate personal struggle—some of the keenest scientific minds, men themselves trained in the art of giving the best counsel. They knew all the answers. Yet these answers, short of the power of God, were totally inadequate for their own needs. The only ladder that could bring these men out of tangled, bitter confusion was the insight, the commitment, the surrender that made the cross of Christ its center and its power.

Christ in the home. This is the ideal. But in spite of the recent surge of religious interest, we are reaping the harvest of a generation of moral abandon, a generation of release from restraint and taboo. For a taboo, we were told, stunted the personality. And so the Ten Commandments were tossed aside as out of date. They just didn't fit into our so-called progressive thinking. Our morals stretched like rubber bands.

Then openly published Kinsey reports and the like convinced us that we were not so bad after all. And psychologists, psychiatrists, and ministers have been overworked ever since.

Is it any wonder that marriages today burn briefly like a paper chain and then are gone?

"Till death do us part." The secret of happiness in marriage is not difficult or profound. Turn back the pages; listen again to the charge on that wedding day as the minister repeated:

"I charge you both that if you wish your new estate to be touched with perennial beauty, cherish those gracious visions which have made springtime within your hearts during the days of your courtship. You must never forget nor deny the vision you once saw; you must resolve that it be not blotted out nor blurred by the commonplace experiences of life. Faults may appear which were once hidden in a golden mist; excellencies may seem to fade in the glare of the noonday sun. Still be unmoved in your devotion; still remain confident and hopeful. Amid the reality of present imperfections believe in the ideal. You saw it once, and it still exists."

What has happened? In a shocking number of cases the ideal is forgotten, and divorce stands at the doorstep. Somewhere along the line the sacred confidence of the family circle has been broken. That moral reserve and dignity that cause the careless and the loose to keep their place have been lost. Advances have been made, hearts broken.

And you don't have to look very far for the root of the trouble. For down in the heart of those discarded Ten Commandments is a very reasonable warning which, if obeyed through the power of God, would guard the purity of the race: "Thou shalt not commit adultery."

However relaxed the moral fabric of the society in which we live, however benumbing the repeated assertion that everybody does it, however convincing the published reports of moral decadence with which we subconsciously compare ourselves, still, God says, "Thou shalt not commit adultery."

Whatever advice may have been given you to the contrary, the Creator of man's body, his mind and emotions, the God who understands our fears and our frustrations and our needs—it is He who says, "Thou shalt not commit adultery."

God calls it adultery. Many, today, call it a meaningful relationship. Any behavior is said to be all right if you call it love. And you decide what to call it while in the grip of an emotional situation.

Only occasionally does a lone voice like that of David Redding come through. He says, "Proponents of the new morality claim that the commandments may be broken in order to fulfill the higher law of love. True, the Christian idea is to do the unique will of God for each special situation. But God never needs to sacrifice principles to satisfy any situation. If we try to keep the commandments even when they appear most inappropriate, God always comes through. . . . The laws stand and perhaps are most in force when we feel least sure. What are any laws good for except for those very occasions when we are being most tempted to abandon them? This God who thinks of everything . . . tailors His laws beautifully to every situation. And if we can hang on to the commandments at the fiery moment when we are certain that keeping them will ruin us, God will do His amazing part, just as He did for Daniel standing that night in the lions' den."—*The New Immorality,* pages 58, 59.

Are the restrictions of God's moral code unreasonable? Is there no better way to rediscover the thrill of living than to fall into some stupid adultery?

There's the problem. How can a man expect marriage to succeed if he has destroyed the barrier that the Creator Himself has placed around it? Can he carelessly ignore the first indiscretion, and not expect a flood of infidelity to come in?

Listen. The breakup of a marriage doesn't happen all at once. It begins with the first neglect of the little attentions that make happiness for a companion. It begins the day you are too tired to be kind, too busy to be thoughtful, too occupied with your own problems to be interested in those of your mate.

Infidelity doesn't happen all at once. The act of adultery is a blow from which the home may never recover. But much has gone before. Infidelity begins when first the relationships of home become routine and dull. Infidelity begins when a man begins to shift his interests from an evening at home to an evening at the shop. Infidelity begins when the husband begins to compare his wife's beauty with that of another, or when she begins to compare her husband's success with that of another. Infidelity begins when he or she first questions the wisdom of their marriage.

Infidelity begins in an unguarded moment. It ends in a betrayal that can forever shatter the confidence of the one you promised to love and cherish.

In answering a question of the Pharisees, our Lord made His position on the matter of divorce and remarriage very clear. Let me read from Dr. Phillip's translation of Matthew 19:3-9:

"Then the Pharisees arrived with a test question. 'Is it right,' they asked, 'for a man to divorce his wife on any grounds whatever?'

" 'Haven't you read,' He answered, 'that the One who created them from the beginning made them male and female and said: *"For this cause shall a man leave his father and mother, and shall cleave to his wife; and the twain shall become one flesh"*? So they are no longer two separate people but one. No man therefore must separate what God has joined together.'

" 'Then why,' they retorted, 'did Moses command us to give a written divorce notice and dismiss the woman?'

" 'It was because you knew so little of the meaning of love that Moses allowed you to divorce your wives! But that was not the original principle. I tell you that anyone who divorces his wife on any grounds except her unfaithfulness and marries some other woman commits adultery.' "

Have you noticed the ease with which some rationalize around the difficulty in order to exchange mates? Yet from what we have read it is clear that the trivial excuses some use could scarcely stand the test of Scripture. Jesus gives us the one situation in which a man or a woman is free to remarry. It is simply this—when he or she discovers himself to be the innocent party in a moral fall.

Love, of course, will do all within its power to forgive and restore. It will not grasp at the sin of a mate as a welcome opening for release. For a divorce, however legitimate, not only seriously mars your own life but tragically undermines the lives of your children.

How often a couple will say, "We think our marriage may go on the rocks. But after all, that is definitely *our* business."

No, friend. Marriage is everybody's business. Each divorce, it is estimated, touches forty or fifty lives. It is a nation's business. Every time a home is destroyed, the whole nation suffers a tremor. It is the child's business. The child, like a seismograph, registers every marital quake. It is God's business, because He wanted to use your love, father and mother, to explain His own love to a child. And now He can't!

"Pastor Vandeman," someone says, "I was divorced and remarried a number of years ago. I didn't consider it seriously then. Most all of our friends were doing it. I'm not sure who was the more innocent or the more guilty, for I didn't care. What shall I do about it now?"

The Word of God has an answer for that sincere inquiry. However serious your marital mixup, please know that if you are deeply and sincerely repentant, you have a God who forgives. "Though your sins be as scarlet, they shall be as white as snow; though they be red like crimson, they shall be as wool." Isaiah 1:18. And this in 1 John 1:9: "If we confess our sins, he is faithful and just to forgive us our sins, and to cleanse us from all unrighteousness."

The Lord has a wonderful way of dealing with matters like this. But though He forgives, though He never condemns, He always adds, "Go, and sin no more."

But however wonderful this provision, I think you can see how God must feel about the man who searches the rules of the church, any church, to discover how he might have his own way and yet continue in good standing. Friend, if this is your reasoning, please be doubly sure that you are testing your own motives as well as the rules of the church.

May I speak for a moment about the innocent one in a situation involving a moral fall? Is it not possible for an individual to be so selfish, so unattentive, so unloving, so downright cold in his or her relationship to his mate that these unfeeling actions make temptation tragically real and all but force the unconsecrated heart to sin?

Oh yes, as far as the church is concerned, he or she may be the innocent party. But one wasn't willing to love, one wasn't willing to lay selfishness aside, to win and hold that mate by true affection. Does not that individual share in the guilt?

Friend, is it possible that an attitude of Pharisaic criticism, even though unexpressed, may be destructive to the very one you most want to help? Listen to the words of Dr. Paul Tournier.

"Every judgment that I make of a man, even if I am careful to say nothing to him, even if I hide it deep in my heart, and even if I am almost or entirely unaware of it myself, makes between him and me an unbridgeable gulf and hopelessly prevents my giving him any effective assistance. By my judgment, I drive him more deeply into his faults rather than free him from them."—*Guilt and Grace,* page 80.

These are the words of a distinguished physician and counselor. They apply not only to marriage but to every human relationship. Dr. Tournier continues: "Thus the most tragic consequence of our criticism of a man is to block his way to humiliation and grace, precisely to drive him into the mechanisms of self-justification and into his faults instead of freeing him from them. For him, our voice drowns the voice of God. We put him beyond the reach of the divine voice which can only be heard in the silence. The impassioned response which our criticism triggers off in his soul makes too much noise."

Have you ever been guilty? I have.

Criticism is destructive anywhere. And when it touches marriage, I think you can see how easy it is to drive that first wedge of hidden blame that eventually separates two hearts. Remember, the ruin of a marriage is not always a dramatic affair. There need be no unfaithfulness, no blows, no desertion. It may be just a slow accumulation of dissatisfactions, a gradual growth of misunderstandings and irritations and petty criticisms until one or the other asks himself, "Did I marry the wrong person?"—and feels wicked for thinking it! At last comes the day when one says, "I can't stand it any longer!" And the other is stunned!

No man or woman can be too careful in guarding the sacred circle of marriage. Once broken, it is difficult to repair.

But however frustrated and confused a life partnership may have become, however futile may seem your efforts at reconciliation of hearts that have grown cold, please remember that divorce should never be thought of as simply a convenient back door out of an unpleasant situation. Divorce cannot heal. No legal or material device, however ingenious, can heal. Only unselfish love and the power of the living Christ can heal. And forgiveness—forgiveness strong enough to say, "I leave the past behind and with hands outstretched to whatever lies ahead I go straight for the goal." Philippians 3:13, 14, Phillips.

How to Escape an Affair

Once upon a time, Cathy and Bill were in love. Now that love is gone. They're not sure when and how it happened, but some how the fire flickered low.

Being unfaithful to Bill had never entered Cathy's mind. At least not till now. She wouldn't admit it even to her best friend, but she can't seem to get that other man off her mind.

Torn between her feelings and her conscience, Cathy wonders, What does this overwhelming temptation mean? A new beginning? Or the end of everything?

And what should she do about it?

You have just met Cathy and Bill. Actually, you've known them for some time. Perhaps they live next door. Or they sing in your church choir. Maybe they even live in your home—*you* might be struggling right now to save your marriage from a crippling affair.

How quickly holy wedlock can become unhappy deadlock! One discouraged husband was reminded by his pastor that he had married for better or for worse. "Yes," the man replied, "but she is worse than I took her for!" And he gave her up to look for someone "better."

It's no secret that adultery has become a national epidemic. Surveys insist that 30 to 50 percent of wives have been unfaithful to their husbands.

For men the situation is even worse. According to the Hite Report on Male Sexuality, 72 percent who have been married two years or longer have committed adultery. Evidently in some states more men cheat than vote!

Shocking statistics indeed! And very sad. But not hopeless! There's hope and help in Jesus to escape an affair. Your marriage can be born again.

Before we discuss God's plan to save your home, let's look in on several stories of struggles married people face. Names and pictures have been changed, but the problems are very real.

Consider Linda's affair with John. She didn't really care about sex. She only craved affection. So she forsook her insensitive husband to be the queen of John's castle. John used adultery to declare his independence. He exchanged a suffocating life with his nagging wife to be refreshed by Linda.

Then there's Jerry and Lisa. Jerry's wife gained a lot of weight after the birth of their first child. And she seemed more interested in caring for the baby than for him. That's when Jerry decided to chase Lisa, a single girl, lonely and vulnerable.

And finally, Bob and Karen. Bob, an attorney in his late forties, worried about growing older. Seeking some way to regain his youth, he flirted with younger women. His secretary, Karen, responded to his advances. Tired of her reckless and immature spouse, she felt drawn like a magnet to Bob. Their affair seemed to meet each other's emotional needs.

These stories could go on and on. Each experience is different, but one fact we will notice remains the same: adultery doesn't solve problems. It compounds them. It's not an oasis but a mirage, unable to quench the thirst for love.

Now let's take another look at the couples we just met.

Linda discovered John's apartment was a dungeon, not a castle. His sweet nothings proved to be just that. John learned Linda could nag as much as his wife. And her cooking was awful.

Jerry also became tired of his affair. He had invested too much in his family to forsake them now. This left Lisa lonelier than ever, abandoned by Jerry's empty promises.

Karen and Bob's secret affair soared through summertime, but fluttered down to earth with autumn's leaves. Satisfied that he could attract a younger woman, Bob no longer needed to prove anything with his secretary. So he left Karen to go home.

Bob's insulted wife demanded he fire his ex-lover. Devastated, Karen attempted suicide.

These heartbreaking experiences follow the same pattern. First those wildly exciting dates on moonlit nights. Then gradually the intoxication wears off. Usually it takes between three and six months to sober up.

You see, people can appear perfect to each other when not sharing the stresses and strains of life. Then sooner or later the real world intrudes and the party's over. Cinderella becomes disenchanted and dissatisfied. Prince Charming gets abrasive or abusive. Fairy tales of romance result in nightmares of regret and the new beginning becomes the end of everything.

Has this been your experience? I have good news for you. There's hope at the end of your rope. Our Father in heaven specializes in rescuing shipwrecked love boats. In His Word we'll discover how your marriage can be born again.

We find a plain and simply warning: "You shall not commit adultery." Exodus 20:14, NKJV.

Our world offers plenty of excuses for indulging in adultery. But the Bible doesn't. No matter what the circumstances, adultery is always inappropriate. Unfaithfulness is a sin. A sin against God. He created our bodies to be the temple of His Holy Spirit.

Adultery also wrongs our spouse. It violates that sacred covenant you made together. Remember your promise. You promised faithfulness to your partner, for better or for worse, as long as you both shall live. And you made that vow at God's sacred altar. Don't take it lightly.

Do you have children? Adultery threatens their homelife and spoils their security. And think of the example set by your disloyalty.

Adultery even harms your illicit lover. Whether married or not, your new partner is bound for heartache sooner or later. He or she doesn't need the spill at the end of the thrill.

Adultery also hurts someone else. Yourself. Because it's suicide. A time bomb of guilt and shame to shatter your peace of mind. And your reputation. Maybe your career. Not to mention the financial and legal hardships from breaking up your home.

No wonder the Bible tells us: "There is a way that seems right to a man, but its end is the way of death." Proverbs 16:25, NKJV.

Adultery may seem all right at first, but it ends in death. The death of your home. The death of your self-respect. And unless you repent, the death of your soul.

Please, don't forget it. Sin may be exciting. But it's also deadly. Fantasy can be fatal.

But take courage. You may be so disappointed and disgusted with yourself that you can't stand the face in your mirror—but the Lord Jesus Christ loves you just the same. Sinful though we are, we may come boldly to our God for mercy. There's plenty enough to erase every one of our sins!

And Jesus offers more than forgiveness. He has power to help us too. You see, He's the Great Physician, the Healer of our hearts and our homes. He doesn't just pity our shame—He can restore us to a new life of respectability.

Are you tempted? Jesus wants to help you just when you need it most. Come boldly to His throne and get inner strength to overcome the most vicious temptation.

Let's make this very practical. You've decided to return to your marriage vows. You know Jesus loves you and longs to help. But how can you receive His power to escape your affair?

First there must be commitment. Give your life to God. Then rededicate yourself to your spouse.

One repenting husband observed, "I had been looking outside the relationship for solutions to our problems. Absurd as it sounds, I found it easier to go to bed with someone else than to talk with my wife. Now I've put my whole heart into working things out at home."

You may need the help of a Christian counselor. Whatever it takes, I urge you to do it! Now, before it's too late.

Maybe you're too discouraged to try working things out. You see no future for your marriage. But believe me—it's amazing how God can heal your home once He has your commitment.

It may not happen overnight. Like everything else in the Christian life, faithfulness in marriage means lifelong effort.

Do what you can to avoid temptation. Quit flirting. Dispose of pornography and all those dreamy novels.

Of course marriage isn't easy. And why should it be? After all, marriage is a ministry. A special calling from God to serve the needs of your partner. Jesus set the example by coming to this earth to serve others, not to be served.

Unselfishness isn't natural for us. I know this from personal experience! We harbor all kinds of expectations of each other. We want our spouse to perform for our pleasure. Girls dream of finding their perfect man. Young men want a Miss America who can cook like Betty Crocker. But God has a better idea. He suggests we drop our checklists and simply love each other.

Who could ever forget that bright January morning in Washington, D.C., when John Kennedy became our president? Remember his stirring inaugural advice: "Ask not what your country can do for you, but rather ask what you can do for your country"? Let's apply this wisdom to your marriage. "Ask not what your spouse can do for you, but rather ask what you can do for your spouse."

Nothing we can do is greater than forgiving each other. And nothing is more challenging. Especially when adultery strikes your home. If you're the victim of your spouse's affair, you may find yourself seething with resentment.

Like the husband who prayed long and earnestly after he learned of his wife's unfaithfulness. He recounted again the betrayal that threatened his home. But over against it were the words of the apostle, "And be kind to one another, tenderhearted, forgiving one another, just as God in Christ also forgave you." Ephesians 4:32, NKJV.

Finally his prayer was answered. He went to his personal safe and took out a sheaf of letters. Here was costly evidence against her loyalty—evidence that might have set him free. He had kept these letters against the day when he might use them in court.

But now God had forgiven his own sin, and he was willing to cast hers into the fire. As the evidence went up in smoke, he saw disappearing all means of getting even. He saw consumed in flame the whip that he had held over his mate's head. Here had been a weapon to destroy. But in one quick moment the condemning words had been transformed into ashes. He was free now—free to forgive!

Forgiveness isn't a feeling. Love itself is more than a feeling. Mother may not feel like jumping out of bed at midnight to nurse a sick child. But love makes her do it anyway. Father doesn't feel like rising before dawn to go to work. But he goes anyway of his own free will—simply because he loves his family.

Perhaps we need to reexamine what it means to be in love. Many couples divorce because they think they have to. Because they've lost that loving feeling, they feel they can't go on together.

How mistaken can we be! You don't have to live by your feelings. You can choose to serve the needs of your spouse from your own free will, no matter how you feel. That's love.

The greatest act of love ever seen is the sacrifice of Jesus on Calvary. Did Christ feel like being nailed to the cruel cross? Did He enjoy hanging in open shame before the mocking mob? No! Not at all.

The night before Jesus died, He agonized alone in the garden of Gethsemane. As bloody sweat poured down His brow, His breaking heart cried, "Father, if it's possible, take this cup of suffering away! If I can save them without going through hell, deliver Me!" But no. His death must be the price of our eternal life. So He pressed on to Golgotha even though every fiber of His being screamed No. He sacrificed His life because He loved us—even though He didn't feel like it.

Suppose you're still not sure you want to stop your affair. Despite the guilt, you have been having a good time—you do not feel like spoiling the party. Then consider Jesus. Remember how your sins broke His heart. Once you understand what your sins cost the Saviour, sinning can never be quite the same.

Even after you end your affair, you may feel more affection for your ex-lover than for your spouse. Your heart may be torn with silent grief. God understands. Feeling or no feeling, invest your emotional energies into your marriage. Put your fantasies to work in pleasing your spouse. Plan special times to be close together, away from the pressures of daily routine. And believe it or not, one day feelings for your spouse can return.

I read somewhere of a young father who had wandered away from God. He had reached the end of his rope. He thought of suicide. Then God touched his life, and he began a new relationship with his family.

He had a boy who was not doing well in school. He had begun to steal things around the neighborhood to gain attention. He was lonely and rebellious. After only two weeks the boy said to his father, "Dad, what's happened to you lately?" The father said slowly, reaching for the right words, "Well, son, I guess I was making a pretty big mess of my life, and I decided I'd ask God to take over and show me how to live it."

The boy looked down at the floor. "Dad," he said quietly, "I think I'd like to do that too."

The father stood there with tears running down his cheeks, and he and the boy wept together. The next day the father left for New York on a business trip lasting two weeks.

He was anxious to get home. When his plane taxied up to the terminal, his son broke through the crowd and ran out to meet his father. His eyes were bright with excitement. "Dad," he said breathlessly, his voice full of wonder, "do you know what God has done?"

"No, son. What has He done?"

"He's changed every kid in my class!"

Friend, God can change every heart in your home. And He can do it now!

Trouble With the Personnel

A young man asked a physician for the hand of his daughter in marriage. The doctor refused. It was quite a setback, but the young suitor gathered courage to ask, "Why can I not marry your daughter? I love her."

The doctor replied, "I think you do."

"I can support her."

"I suppose you can."

"Then why can't I marry her?"

To this the doctor answered, "My daughter has a miserable disposition. Nobody could live with her and be happy."

The young man gallantly replied, "But there is always the grace of God."

The doctor smiled understandingly. "When you are as old as I am, young man, you will realize that the grace of God can live with some people that you can't live with!"

The trouble with marriage is not with the institution. It's with the personnel. The trouble is with people. It's people that need to be changed. Unhappy couples don't dislike marriage. They dislike each other. The challenge in marriage is not only in *finding* the right person, but *being* the right person. Many a wife has thought she needed a new husband, only to realize that her husband needed a new wife.

Too many marriages have gone on the rocks because one partner entered the contract secretly planning to change the other. And it doesn't usually work that way. If a bus says "Cincinnati," that is likely where it is going. You can't count on its changing destinations after you board it. It's the same with husbands and wives.

Glenn Clark, popular author and publisher, has listed some beatitudes of a happy marriage. One of them is this: "Blessed are the married ones who strive first of all to make their mates *happy* rather than *good*."

The trouble is that so many of us feel it is our duty to make our mates good—and we sometimes make everyone concerned unhappy in the process. I have been guilty. But I have discovered that if we persevere in trying to make our mates happy, we more easily succeed in the other objective.

We are talking here about sound principles of interpersonal relationship. To be sure, they are especially applicable in the unique relationships of marriage where a home must survive or perish. But the same foundation principles will succeed in the relations of friend with friend, doctor with patient, employer with employee. And surprisingly enough, we often discover that the difficulty is not *between* two people, but *within* two people, *within* the individual. Changing your own heart, you see, is likely to be the surest and fastest way to change the heart of your mate.

Why do we continue to struggle with the simplest lessons in personal relations when we ought to be taking an advanced course? One couple visited a marriage counselor after nineteen years of marriage. The counselor told them, "You have not had nineteen years of experience in marriage. You have simply lived the first year nineteen times."

The secrets of marital success are not elusive. I feel strongly that if we would put the hard work and ingenuity into our homes that we put into our jobs, we would succeed.

Tact and insight. These are invaluable in the office environment. They are equally indispensable at home. Human nature does not respond charitably to bluntness. Tact, you see, is saying the right thing, the right kind of thing, at the right time, in the right way. Tact involves not only words, but the tone of voice, the mood, the atmosphere, the motive. And insight is the willingness to understand another's point of view—with the possibility that it may be right. Together they are the healing therapy that reaches into a wounded heart and avoids a crisis. Without tact and insight, marriage often becomes a contest in which each partner tries to wound more deeply than the other.

Why should we be so blind to the fact that we have faults too? The most ideal person has faults. And marriage in itself does not eliminate them. But we get in a hurry. We expect marriage to solve automatically and instantly all the problems we had before marriage.

A college girl knows that it takes time to adjust to a new roommate. A violinist knows that he will not be a professional when first he picks up the instrument. But we expect marriage to be different. We may be unhappy single. We may be miserable in school. We may be in conflict with our parents. But we expect marriage to change us miraculously and instantaneously into ecstatically happy persons. And it doesn't work that way.

It is when we begin to accept life as it is, and our mates as they are, that we begin to move toward a happy home.

A young wife, married about three years, breezed into her pastor's office, tossed her coat over a chair, and exploded, "Honestly, Bill is the most ornery, stubborn, independent, obstinate—ooooh! But you know what? I'm learning to live with him! Now how do you like that?" And then she added, "He's adorable! I would never have believed it possible that I could be so extremely exasperated with a man yet love him so dearly." And she was gone.

Of course, if you are normal, you have probably experienced some degree of marital tension. There are those who say they have never quarreled. That may be true. Or it may be that they are simply giving their quarrels another label. One husband said, "We've never had an argument in thirty years of married life. However, we have engaged in serious discussions which the neighbors heard a block away."

Every home, I say, has some problems. Some homes more than others. A marriage counselor asked one young couple, "What do you have in common?"

The wife replied, "One thing. Neither of us can stand the other."

John Milton, the unhappily married poet, once heard his wife referred to as a rose. He remarked, "I am no judge of flowers. But it may be true, for I feel the thorns daily." And John Wesley's wife used to sit in City Road Chapel and make faces at him while he preached!

Let me repeat again, there are no good quarrels. It is unfortunate that those who write the marriage manuals often think it necessary to include a chapter on how to quarrel. Don't we agree that quarrels only weaken the relationship, each encounter leaving it less secure?

There was the man who said, "Oh, she would never leave me."

"Don't be too sure," said the minister to whom the wife had already come in great distress.

And the man said, "Why, she can't do that to me. What would I do without her?"

The minister asked quietly, "Did you ever tell her that?"

"No," the man admitted. "I don't like such talk."

When it was suggested that he take home some flowers and recourt the woman of his choice, this huge, clumsy-looking fellow exclaimed, "Now wouldn't I look fine luggin' home flowers? I'd feel like a fool." Just the same, he did it. And it broke the growing coolness, stimulated the basic, strong, original affection between them.

Too simple to work, you say? Don't you believe it. Flowers may not always be the answer. But a lack of appreciation in small things can eventually grow until it becomes a great divisive factor.

Do you take your mate for granted? Or are you attempting, by little acts of thoughtfulness, coupled with the appropriate words, to protect your marriage against deterioration? Is your companion secure in your affection? Does she know, does he know, that no attack from without can shake the ship of matrimony? Do the children know it?

One expert has said, "The most important thing a father can do for his children is to love their mother." How quickly little children are unsettled by dissension in the home! Only when they know that nothing can crack the rock of their domestic tranquility will they be content.

Do you remember—even in moments of crisis—that your wife is a person—your children are persons? Do you remember their need for a sense of security and a feeling of personal worth? Have you made a determined effort to understand those needs? For tragedy sets in, homes begin to disintegrate, when we do not understand. It starts with little neglects, little misunderstandings, little selfish attitudes—until finally there is constant bulldozing and belittling until the last spark of identity is killed and the heart is drained of its desire to continue!

Nagging, that demonic tactical maneuver in a psychological battle, is often the culprit. Said the wise man, "A continual dripping on a rainy day and a contentious woman are alike." Proverbs 27:15, RSV.

And one modern authority says, "Most cases of emotionally induced illness are the result of a monotonous drip, drip of . . . unpleasant emotions, the everyday run of anxieties, fears, discouragements and longings."—Dr. John Schindler, *How to Live 365 Days a Year,* page 13.

Who can take the drip-of-the-faucet treatment for long—especially when it comes from someone you love?

How can the rift be healed? How can the gulf be bridged? Communication. That is the answer. Talking it over is a cornerstone in building a successful marriage. There should be a willingness to talk at all times. Many a misunderstanding could be healed in minutes if both partners would calmly evaluate it. There is nothing in all of marriage more destructive than the presence of a silent rift.

One wife said, "You know how you feel when the phone rings and nobody answers? That is how I feel."

There is a lifetime of communication ahead of each of us. Wouldn't it be wise to learn the art better? The heart of marriage is its communication system. Communication breakdown is a chief source of trouble in all human relationships—especially in the intimate and continuing relationship of marriage.

It is impossible not to communicate. If we do not communicate with words, we will be communicating by our silence. And our silence may be as easily misunderstood as our words.

The communication in marriage is not the same as communication of courtship. The excitement of exploring each other's lives begins to disappear. The girl who was once so glamorous is now washing dishes. The ability to communicate now, in changing circumstances, may determine whether the marriage survives or not.

Honesty at this point is all-important. Playing games will not do. Wearing masks will not do. Masks cannot communicate. Only people can communicate. And the intimate ties of marriage are never strengthened by pretense.

Those who communicate, in any area of life, face one baffling problem: *Is anyone listening?* Do you hear what your wife says? Or is your mind taking a meaningful excursion elsewhere? It is estimated that we spend about 70 percent of our waking hours in communication of some kind—speaking, listening, reading, or writing. Evidently listening is mighty important.

Marriage, unfortunately, provides no guarantee that the partners will listen to each other, or try to understand each other. Too often when one is speaking, the other is really not present. He is running errands in his mind. The happy lesson to be learned is that love listens. It is only as love listens that love can understand. Listening will do what words cannot. Did you ever try to find the right words to let someone know his opinions are important to you? Listening will do it as if by magic.

Sometimes, in the marital relationship, you get a busy signal. If a husband has been barraged with messages all day, he may, without ever knowing it, tune out his wife just as he would a television set. One wife said, "My husband can have the TV and the radio on at the same time, listening to two different games at once. The kids can pester him endlessly with interruptions, yet he can tell you the progress of either game whenever you ask. This is the same guy who can sit at the supper table without any distractions whatever and not hear a word I say."

Evidently we *choose* to listen.

Human nature is so persistent. Speaking, you see, is a way of asserting one's self. Listening is not. That's why it is easier to speak than to listen. This inward need for self-assertion is manifested in many ways. For instance, there is the chronic interrupter who constantly attempts to take the ball. There is the one who breaks into the conversation with "that reminds me" and diverts the topic of discussion into his own channel. Then there is the one who breaks in with "I know just what you are going to say," and thereby robs the speaker of any opportunity whatever for unique expression. Such a listener listens with only one thought in mind—"Where do I come in?"

Then there is the man who is always right. There can be no productive conversation with him. His mind is already closed. Lucy, of *Peanuts* fame, says, "I have a new ambition. When I get big, I'd like to be a baseball umpire." Charlie Brown asks, "What in the world makes you think you could be a good baseball umpire?" With head high, Lucy replies, "Because I'm always right!"

Excessive talking, which may or may not be compulsive, is another way to avoid listening. Sometimes it is an attempt to divert the conversation from an unwelcome subject. Who has not seen it?

One of the most frequent problems in marriage is the husband who will not listen. But is the conversation worth listening to? The wife should make sure it is. Small talk may seem entirely too insignificant in contrast with the big ideas that have filled the husband's office hours.

Marriage partners who will not listen are already experiencing a separation of interests. For where there is no dialogue, there is emotional divorce. Would it be too strong to suggest that whenever one mate stops listening to the other, he is guilty of a sort of infidelity? It is in attentive and understanding listening that marriage matures.

Talk is absolutely essential in marriage. It's married strangers who quarrel most readily. Silence may be golden—sometimes. But silence can also kill. Buttoned-up lips too often indicate an unsteady heart. Without verbal spillways the tension inside becomes too great, and tragedy can result. The very first barrier to communication should be a danger signal.

One of the most frequent circuit jammers in the marital communication system is the perfectionist within us. The perfectionist is never on a level with his mate. He has to prove everything he says. Even when he is wrong he is right. He may make a good proofreader, but can you think of a more impossible person to live with? Successful marriage partners early learn to communicate as imperfectionists. The apostle John says, "If we say that we have no sin, we deceive ourselves." 1 John 1:8.

I have learned to my chagrin that good communication is deeply involved in semantics.

You know, of course, what a particular word means to you. But what does it mean to your mate? Brittle relationships can be broken by a troublesome word. Is it asking too much for a husband, instead of resorting to stupid adjectives, to say gently, "Why, yes, I can *see* how *anyone* would misunderstand. But this is what I meant."

When a husband and wife get into heated debate, there is always the temptation to forsake the issue and attack the person. There is a Latin term for it—*ad hominem,* meaning "to the man." There are lawyers who, finding themselves without a case, resort to personal attacks. But let's keep the *ad hominems* out of marriage. It's the personal arrows that fly straightest to the mark and leave the deepest scars.

Many a marital rift can be quickly healed by calmly, quietly, and understandingly talking it over. But remember. A sense of security and a feeling of personal worth—these are the basis for opening doors. There can be no useful communication without them. Talking things over without first reestablishing this interrupted undercurrent of confidence in each other's affections is often useless. Communication without first reaffirming one's affection may only degenerate into defense and justification and accusation. Only when love is first solidly reanchored can there be a basis for understanding.

Tell me, Is your antenna so directed that your companion can receive the message? Is yours a relaxed attitude—an environment that encourages talking it over? There may be a torrent of words. But if there is not an attitude of confidence and respect and willingness to listen to the other side with the possibility that it may even be the right side, there is no real communication.

"I love you." These are hard words to say in a moment of tension and misunderstanding. But we need to say them. And we may need to add three words even harder to say—"I was wrong." There are times when a heart cannot be healed without those words. No wonder that the apostle James wrote, "Confess your faults one to another, and pray one for another, that ye may be healed." James 5:16.

You ask, "What does confession have to do with healing?"

Simply this. We are fast learning that fear, anger, resentment, and bitterness not only lay the groundwork for divorce, but actually poison the body system. Fussing one's way to the divorce court also may lead to the hospital. The body is not made for hate. Body, mind, and soul are made for happiness.

We need to remember that a marital rift, with the scars it has left on mind and body, is healed more easily with words of honest confession than with gifts. In fact, one of the serious delusions of our day is the notion that hearts can be mended with material things. We seem to be caught up in a feverish rush to acquire more and more in the elusive hope of finding happiness and understanding therein.

A few years ago a huge floor-covering corporation featured a delightful ad with all the color and modern appeal of design. Across the ad in striking, bold letters were these words: "Lay linoleum and have a happy home!"

Do you see? Too often when there is home trouble, we think we can heal it if we *lay linoleum*. If there is quarreling or bickering, *lay linoleum*. If the children are wild and disobedient, *lay linoleum*. Laying linoleum—or wall-to-wall carpet for that matter, installing a deepfreeze, or contracting for a second automobile—however useful or pleasant, is not the secret of a lasting marriage.

Too many homes are trying to substitute things for words, responsibility for romance, tolerance for love—and hoping the world will never guess!

The late Dr. Louis Evans drew a fascinating lesson from a detail little noticed in the story of ancient Israel. You can read it in 1 Kings 14. Solomon, in the days of his glory, had made "three hundred shields of beaten gold." Then Solomon died, and the glory of the kingdom perished with him.

In the days of Rehoboam, son of Solomon, we read that Shishak, leader of the enemy hosts, "took away all the shields of gold which Solomon had made."

What should they do now? The glory had faded. But Rehoboam determined that the world should never know. He would keep up appearances. He gave the order to make as many shields of brass and shine them until they glittered as pure gold. With these they were to parade bravely and unfalteringly.

"In many a home," says Dr. Evans, "the golden shields of romance have been stolen; the thievery of time or drabness or selfishness or treason or coldness have walked away with the golden shields of romance and rich newness. Marriage is no longer a parade, it is a sullen march."—*Your Marriage—Duel or Duet?* page 123.

How is it in your home, friend? Are you bravely parading with highly polished shields of brass, when they might have been—might still be—shields of pure gold?

What of those who watch the parade? Is your home a convincing demonstration of happiness wall to wall? Do friends and neighbors covet its secret?

And what of the children, the teenagers who are a part of that home? What does it look like from the inside? Gold? Or brass? Do they consider it the genuine thing? Or only a careless copy? Are they using it as a pattern for their own interpersonal relationships? Are they planning to borrow its blueprint for homes of their own? Or are they left to solve the teenage dilemma with shields of brass, a heritage of make-believe?

There is no more important question.

Your Irreplaceable Role

Remember Claude Monet—the revolutionary genius who taught the world to see in a totally different way? The play of light and color on his canvases revolutionized the art world. His exhibitions at first produced shock, outrage, and quiet awe. In time, the world would come to regard him as uniquely inspired. But Claude Monet's talented eye failed to see, really see, one critical thing: a girl named Camille. And she proved to be the one irreplaceable part of his inspiration.

In nineteenth-century Paris, the Academy of Fine Arts was all-powerful. For artists, the road to success lay through Academy teachers who taught painting in the approved style: correct, finished, and lifeless. Talented students might someday exhibit their works in the Academy Salon. Only there could a painter receive the attention of the critics and, eventually, admission to the Academy.

Claude Monet, however, just couldn't bring himself to take that road. What was the point of merely copying the same old scenes in a certain style? Monet had to paint what his own eye saw, directly from nature. He wanted to capture the liveliness of things—the interaction of light, color, and shape in one momentary impression.

Monet's parents wanted to help their son become a great painter. But they insisted that he take the respectable way toward a more prosperous art career. "You must study with the Academy of Fine Arts," they said, "or we will not support you."

This Monet could not do. So he struggled on alone, barely

scraping together enough to live on, and painting, always painting. "I am the prisoner of my eye," he once said. His one unchanging goal would always be to represent truthfully his own vision of life and nature.

One of Monet's favorite subjects was Camille, a beautiful, graceful model. His admiration for her deepened into love, and they were married.

Monet had become a leader in the new art movement called Impressionism. But he could not sell his work. When he exhibited paintings in galleries, the crowds only laughed. The critics were sarcastic. "Even wallpaper . . . is more finished than THAT," one said. A newspaper cartoon pictured a policeman warning pregnant women to stay away from an Impressionist exhibition—the shock would be too great.

Monet and Camille endured much privation. The struggle to get enough food and find a place to stay seemed endless. But Camille never complained. She believed in her husband's dream.

And through worry, disappointment, and suffering, Monet continued to produce his bright, lively canvases. Camille had become central to his art. She appears in many of his paintings—in the fields, tall and stately—in their gardens—on the beach—and with their son Jean. Her deep, dark eyes hint at both sorrow and a quiet determination.

But the strain of barely surviving took its toll. Camille's health was suffering. Monet became desperate. She just had to get better. But how? He couldn't bring himself to stop painting and find some respectable job. Monet felt terribly guilty, but his obsession drove him on.

After the birth of their second child, Camille's illness worsened. Now they knew she had tuberculosis. Monet continued to paint feverishly, hoping against hope for a breakthrough. Surely someone would recognize his work soon; his paintings would sell; they could settle into more comfortable surroundings, and all would be well.

But the breakthrough didn't come in time. In 1879 tuberculosis claimed Camille's life. Monet still had a studio full of unsold paintings. Camille had never complained; she had always supported her husband in his work. But now she was gone.

And something else was lost too, though Monet didn't realize it at first. As one biographer put it, "With Camille's death, his wonderful eye lost its most powerful creative force." All the warmth, the humanity, and the deep feeling in his pictures had come, indirectly, from her.

A few years later the breakthrough finally arrived. The public had begun to accept Impressionism. Monet's paintings started to sell. His reputation grew. Finally Monet was making it as an artist—but without Camille. Monet was tortured by this thought: Could even the struggle for true art be worth the life of such a woman?

Monet was selling his older paintings, but he had difficulty with new work. He wrote, "I have scraped off all my latest canvases. I suffer anguish." And later in another location he said, "I've destroyed six [canvases] since coming here. I've done only one that pleases me. I'm tired of it all."

Monet had only to paint what he pleased, and it would sell for any price he demanded. But he found himself increasingly bitter and restless. "I work hard," he wrote, "and make myself ill with wretchedness: I'm horribly worried by everything I do."

Monet had lost the one irreplaceable part of his inspiration. He had reason to be bitter, but perhaps he also had reason to reconsider. Monet had sacrificed his wife for his art, and then discovered that there could be little meaningful art without her. Monet's brilliant eye had not quite seen that Camille herself was his art and that making compromises to better care for her would have better preserved his art as well.

His admirable pursuit of excellence in art had not included a drive to be excellent at home—at the root of his inspiration.

Many of us have a similar problem. It is not always easy to balance the demands of our mission, our profession, with the needs of our home. We don't always see clearly what is truly irreplaceable. Tom was fortunate enough to make that discovery before it was too late.

Tom worked as a television technician. He was often called on to assist in the taping of special events. Tom was proud of his work; he understood the intricacies of television electronics well and had developed a special talent for troubleshooting during taping sessions.

One year Tom's union and the company he worked for couldn't settle on a contract. The union called a strike. Tom, along with the rest of his crew, walked off the job.

Tom didn't like the idea of just quitting. He felt uneasy sitting around the house. But he felt sure the company would settle on a contract quickly. After all, how could they get along without him and his crew? After years of experience, Tom had learned almost every detail involved in the production of a television program. Who else could they get with his expertise?

The strike, however, dragged on. The company didn't seem that desperate to compromise. And then Tom learned that he had been replaced. That was quite a blow—someone else filling his role. And what was worse, the company continued producing programs just as before. Tom had become dispensable.

His spirits plummeted. If he could be replaced so easily, how much did his life mean—what purpose could he really have? He wandered about the house aimlessly. But during this time of depression, Tom's family rallied around him. They comforted and encouraged him.

It was then that he began seeing himself in a new light. He looked again at those who depended on him day by day—his wife and children. And it dawned on Tom that there was one role in life no one but he could fulfill. There was one place where he would always be irreplaceable: in his family.

If Tom, the husband and father, went out on strike, no replacement would ever be found. No one else could have the same nurturing relationships he enjoyed with his wife and children.

Tom eventually went back to work and continued a productive career in television. But he no longer depended on his position for security. He understood where he was truly irreplaceable.

Have you made that discovery? Are you committed to fulfilling your one irreplaceable role? Or does your career crowd out time with the family? Does the pursuit of a promotion take priority over caring for your wife or husband?

Oh, I know we all give lip service to the idea that our families are most important. That's easy to SAY. But ask yourself this: When a decision has to be made between a demand at work and a need at home, how often do you choose the latter? Do you ever cancel appointments because you need to spend time with the family?

Probably not very often. Believe me, I know. We ministers are often the worst offenders—so busy trying to save the world that we neglect those closest to us.

The God of the Bible, however, has a different view of the matter. He values most what we often pass over. God made that point beautifully in a little book called Ruth. At the beginning of this Old Testament story we find three widows trudging down the long road from Moab to Judah. They are Naomi and her two daughters-in-law, Ruth and Orpah. A famine has been ravaging Moab. And Naomi has decided to go back to Judah, where food is more plentiful.

But as she walks on the dusty road, Naomi begins to think. Ruth and Orpah, both Moabites, will never be able to marry in Judah. As foreigners they will never be fully accepted. The girls would be better off staying in Moab. At least among their own people they *have* a chance of raising a family.

So Naomi stops and tells them, "Go back, each of you, to your mother's home. May the Lord show kindness to you."

But Ruth and Orpah reply, "We will go back with you to your people." After all, they are all the elderly woman has left. How could she survive alone?

Naomi, however, is insistent: "Return home, my daughters. Why would you come with me? Am I going to have any more sons, who could become your husbands?" Ruth 1:8-11, NIV.

Finally, Orpah embraces her mother-in-law and says a tearful farewell. But Ruth just can't tear herself away. Her devotion is too strong. This young girl makes a memorable promise: "Where you go I will go, and where you stay I will stay. Your people will be my people and your God my God. Where you die I will die." Ruth 1:16, 17, NIV.

Beautiful words. I can't imagine a more eloquent loyalty.

Ruth understood her one irreplaceable role. She committed herself to the one family bond that remained.

Just two people, clinging to each other on the long road to Judah. You might think they would be rather insignificant in the vast sweep of biblical history. But God has emphasized their story. Ruth plays a special part in God's revelation. The book is actually His exclamation point at the end of another book called Judges.

Judges tells a pretty sorry story of Israel's repeated apostasies. At times, after some great deliverance, Israel would return to God, but soon they would be running after their neighbor's idols again. They could never decide altogether for the God of heaven.

Ruth is God's answer to that whole sad period. What a contrast this heathen girl provides to Israel's wishy-washy ways! God didn't need to preach a long sermon on loyalty after Israel's disappointing performance under the judges. He just told this beautiful story of a girl and her mother-in-law.

This is what is really significant, God is saying. Kings and warriors may come and go, nations pass through prosperity and disaster, but this kind of loyal relationship is what matters in the end.

Ruth valued, above all, the role no one else could fill. And as a result she became one of God's great signs in history.

Your marriage can be another of God's beautiful signs. Paul tells us that the relationship between husband and wife is to reflect the relationship between Christ and His church. The world must see, in the care, consideration, and respect of our home life, a picture of Christ's love for His people.

Nothing in our work, nothing in our careers, can provide that picture. All the marketing and advertising and salesmanship in the world can't provide it. Only the quality of our marriage relationships can say what God wants to say. We have an irreplaceable role to play.

God wants us to excel in our relationships at home. It is all part of our calling. It can't be separated from our mission in life. If we sacrifice our families for our mission, we will find, like the painter Monet, that we have no mission left.

Excellence in our family relationships—how few of us seek it. The pressures of the world constantly seek to divorce our calling at work from our calling at home.

Recently hundreds of academic professionals gathered to honor a man who had earned a Nobel prize in science. During the preliminary ceremonies his wife waited backstage with the wives of other men also to be honored. The wife of the Nobel prize winner didn't seem all that excited, and the other women asked her why.

"How can I be happy with a husband like that?" she asked, and went on to describe a rather pathetic home life.

Immediately the other women chimed in, "Why, that's my story, exactly." All had the same experience of neglect and abuse.

While cameras flashed on the stage and dignitaries gave admiring speeches, a very different story was unveiled backstage. Those closest to the honorees could only describe a common misery.

Excelling at work and failing at home. That's the status quo. And that's what the Word of God will not tolerate. Our mission in life is one seamless fabric. If we can't reflect Christ in our home life, what is the point of trying to promote Him at our jobs?

But I believe each of us *can* excel in our marriage relationships. Columnist Judith Viorst found the following choice gems of excellence in marriage. These show that acts of thoughtful love are not often dramatic. No bands are playing or crowds applauding. It is the quiet, thoughtful, gracious acts which make families great.

Excellence starts with a commitment to take time. Elsa and Steve were arguing at breakfast one weekday morning. Their animated discussion continued as Steve brushed his teeth and dressed for work. He was about to walk out the door when Elsa cried, "How can you just go off like that! We haven't settled a thing!"

Steve stared at his wife a moment. He was an ambitious and highly motivated executive. But he stopped, walked to the phone, and cancelled all his appointments for that day. Elsa was deeply moved. He had said, in effect, that their relationship meant more than his urgent business meetings.

After we commit ourselves to investing time in our family role, we can begin looking for new ways to express our love. June and Mac had been asked to bring dessert to a buffet supper. Though not an experienced baker, June managed to produce a chocolate custard pie. As they were driving to the party, the couple detected a smell of scorched custard. June began to fear her pie might be totally inedible.

It joined other desserts on the hostess's buffet table. June sliced it and offered her husband a bit. By the horrified look on his face she knew the pie was a disaster.

But Mac grabbed the pie and announced to the guests that since there were so many desserts there, and since this pie happened to be his favorite, he was going to eat it all by himself.

Mac sat in a corner that evening, valiantly eating chocolate custard and mashing up the slices he couldn't get down. No one ever knew how awful it had turned out.

What is true in business is also true in marriage: nothing succeeds like success. Consideration breeds more consideration. Thoughtfulness creates more thoughtfulness. As you take the time to build a good relationship at home, you will find that opportunities for excellence abound.

Jack found one on a freezing, cold night. He quietly sneaked upstairs and warmed up the sheets for his wife by ironing them.

When Helen's depressed husband accidentally burned a hole in their new window-seat cover, she embroidered a colorful flower over the charred spot—and inspired her husband with hope.

Fred was forbidden to be with his terrified wife at the birth of their baby. But he found a way into the delivery room—disguised as an orderly.

All these people found ways to excel in the one role no one else can fulfill. Their acts of consideration demonstrated Christ's love. They are God's signs in the world.

Angie and David's home burned to the ground soon after their sixth anniversary. When they were allowed to look through the blackened remains, Angie's first act was to search for their precious photo albums. When she went to tell David that the pictures had survived, she found him kneeling in the ashes, carefully placing in a box their courtship love letters.

In that moment Angie realized how much they were meant for each other. In the midst of their greatest tragedy their first thought was not on material loss, but on what might have been lost of their life together.

Angie and David understood well what was irreplaceable. They were among the lucky ones, working to preserve what really matters.

How are you doing in your irreplaceable role? When our world turns to ashes, we will not look back and say, "I wish I'd spent more time in the office." We will only look at the quality of our personal relationships. Our keenest joys and deepest regrets will all center on the people in our family circle we have touched for good or ill.

In this final moment with this chapter, will you be prepared to seek excellence where it really counts? Will you commit yourself to fulfill your irreplaceable role? I hope so.

When Wounds Won't Heal

Small children who fall and scrape their knees usually have Mommy nearby, ready with a band-aid and a kiss to make it all better. Teenagers enduring still another dateless Saturday night can count on a trusted friend to ease the lonely hours. And after marriage, most people find some way of coping with the occasional hurts and disappointments of adulthood.

But what about the wounds that band-aids and comforting words just don't reach? What about the emotional traumas that leave scars deep inside us? What do we do when wounds simply refuse to heal?

Three-year-old Lori is playing happily one day outside her home in a Denver suburb. A young man drives up, parks by the curb, and entices the child into his car. Moments later, Lori's mother notices that the child has disappeared. She begins to search, at first calmly, then frantically, for her missing daughter. The police are notified. They alert personnel all over the city. Lori has disappeared without a trace.

A few days pass. A group of bird watchers are hiking through a mountain park about forty minutes from Lori's home. Suddenly they stop on the trail—somewhere a child is crying. The hikers follow the faint cries to an outhouse. Opening the door, they look down into the pit and see something they will never forget. A child stands in the filth, shivering, almost naked. "What are you doing here?" they ask. "I'm home," little Lori replies. "I live here."

This innocent three-year-old had been sexually abused. Lori

was reunited with her tearful parents—safe at last in her mother's arms. But the wound—the wound would remain.

Was Lori an isolated case? Unfortunately not. We live in a scar-intensive world. Children now must face terrible new facts of life.

Not long ago, the quiet, grandmotherly founder of a Los Angeles preschool was arrested. Authorities charged that she and other staff members had molested more than forty children over the course of a decade. For years the preschool staff had frightened their toddlers into silence by slaughtering small animals in front of them. But finally, with the help of trained counselors, a few of the children managed to tell their horror stories of intimidation and abuse.

Stories of molestation abound, and we learn to our shock that the criminal is often a relative or friend of the family, betraying the trust of an innocent child.

We hear unbelievable accounts of children brutalized by their parents, infants neglected, latch-key kids left to fend for themselves, adolescents kidnapped by pornographers, child prostitutes walking the streets of our great cities.

Ours is by all counts a scar-intensive world. Is it any wonder that so many suffer from damaged emotions?

And these are only the most sensational of the traumas that wound people so deeply. Most of us have had a less-than-perfect past, and many of us are burdened with some hidden scar—a secret wound that never quite heals.

Many things can scar. A parent who could never quite accept our performance—we were never quite good enough. Classmates who teased us unmercifully at some awkward, vulnerable age. A friend who betrayed us in an hour of need. An old sin that keeps gnawing away at our souls.

When traumas in our past produce emotional scars, our self-esteem is often damaged. We feel inadequate and try to make up for this lack in a number of unhealthy ways.

First, many of us try to hide from our scars. We try to ignore them and pretend that the wounds simply don't exist. It's so very hard to accept the fact that something terrible—something very unjust—has happened to us.

But scars, though hidden, still can hamper our lives. In running away from them, we get tangled up in emotional detours. Some begin to think, subconsciously, "I must have done something terrible to deserve such a tragedy." A twisted sense of guilt can develop, leading us to say, "No one could ever love me. Everything I do ends up wrong."

Hidden scars sometimes drive people toward a false perfectionism—always trying hard to be good enough, desperately trying to please others. But they never can seem to make it. They never feel good enough; they can never find rest.

Hidden scars can make people supersensitive. They once reached out for approval and love and were deeply wounded. Bearing that hurt inside makes them overly sensitive to further pain. Some walk around with their hearts on their sleeves; others cover up their sensitivity with tough exteriors. In either case, the real wound remains—hidden, unhealed, festering.

Hidden scars make people afraid. At some point in the past they became victims. That experience convinced them that they really can't control what happens to them. And they remain victims. Fears force people to the sidelines. They watch life go by from behind the barrier of their hidden scars.

If you have been deeply wounded, you may feel that nothing can penetrate that barrier and that nothing can undo the emotional damage. You may well think that past traumas will haunt you always.

But I believe there is genuine healing available for the deepest wound. There is a way to deal with our damaged emotions, our wounded self-esteem. There are steps we can take, through God's grace, to gain control of our lives again. Our Lord wants us to be disciples, not simply victims.

First, we must deal with the problem squarely. We must be willing to come face to face with that hidden wound.

Ben had been cowering his way through life, always afraid of attempting anything, always afraid of offending someone. He spoke in a barely audible voice. Something was obviously holding him back. Help finally came at a marriage-enrichment retreat. Surrounded by loving, supporting Christians, he was able to share some painful memories.

When Ben was a boy, his mother had suffered a nervous breakdown. Shortly afterward he overheard the neighbors whispering. "You know why she had a breakdown," they said. "It's because of that little boy, following her around all the time, clinging to her apron strings."

Now that's a pretty heavy burden for a child to carry. Imagine hearing people say, "You are the cause of your mother's breakdown, of her being an invalid." All those years Ben had been doing inner penance for an unjust accusation. He was trying to make up for the terrible wrong he thought he had done.

But as Ben shared with this group, the burden was lifted. As he sobbed out his painful story, he experienced release and acceptance for the first time.

Ben had to face that hidden scar. He had to say, "Yes, it happened. Yes, it was terribly unfair, but I'm going to step through that false accusation; I'm going to say goodbye."

As we are enabled to face our hidden scars, we need to face something else too—our responsibility. Now let me explain. We are not responsible for the trauma in our past. We are not somehow guilty for being wounded. No. But we ARE responsible for our reaction to the hurt. We can take charge of our response.

Let me tell you about Josephine. This deeply troubled young woman insisted, to all her doctors, that she wasn't her father's daughter. She was absolutely certain of it. The records proved otherwise, but nothing could persuade Josephine.

Then a Christian physician began to counsel with her. He discovered that, years before, this woman had been mistreated by her father and had rebelled against his harshness. Gently this physician tried to lead her to a healthier response to her unfortunate past.

It was a hard struggle. Josephine had a difficult time accepting her father. But after much prayer and counsel, she came to realize that her denial only worsened the wounds. She discovered a new fellowship with God and was able to become reconciled to her father.

You see, we must decide whether we really want to recover from our wounds. Do we want to take charge of our response to the past? We must answer the question Jesus posed to the paralytic lying helplessly by the Pool of Bethesda: "Do you want to be healed?"

Jesus didn't ask, "Do you want to lie here and talk about your problem?" or, "Do you want to complain about how unfairly life has treated you?" The Saviour simply asked, "Do you want to be healed?"

Now we come to a very important step. As we accept responsibility for our response to a wound, we must learn to forgive those who have wounded us. And that's not easy. In fact, humanly speaking, it is often impossible.

All our lives we may have been trying to collect on a debt. Someone owes us for the terrible hurt we've experienced. Subconsciously we expect people to pay up.

A Christian scholar found himself reacting in a violent anger at the most unexpected times. He couldn't understand it. The man read the Scriptures, he prayed, but still couldn't quite get a handle on the problem.

Finally, he paid a visit to a Christian counselor. He began recalling incidents from childhood—grade-school sports—how clumsy he had been! Every recess was agony for him. The bigger boys bullied him around. Others made fun of his awkwardness.

Now, years later, those scenes were vivid in his mind. He could recall the faces and names of each of his tormentors. Evidently this was the root of his anger.

So the scholar was led through a simple exercise. He named each of those schoolmates and placed them under God's forgiveness: "I claim forgiveness for Jack, I claim forgiveness for Sally," and so on.

This was painful, but through his prayer the scholar found the grace to truly forgive, and slowly God healed those painful scars of the heart.

Jesus taught that we should forgive one another just as He has forgiven us. Christ forgives freely, without reservation. Forgiveness freely given opens up our hearts for healing.

Now we can bring our feelings to God. Our feelings of anger, humiliation, shame. Feelings we dared not share before. We can bring them to Him because He is the Wounded Healer.

He is the One who sobbed heart and soul out on the cold

ground of Gethsemane. He is the One wounded for our trangressions and bruised for our iniquities, the One rejected by His own people, the One who endured mockery as He hung alone on the cross.

Whatever dark picture stains your memory, He will understand. He has seen darker still. Whatever painful trauma continues to haunt you, He can bear. He has born a greater pain.

Share that secret hurt with a heavenly Father, a Wounded Healer, who sympathizes with your weakness. As you share your pain, He will share His healing grace. And you will be able to accept His regard, His picture of who you really are. God has a lot to say about whom we really are.

Listen to the apostle John's exclamation: "How great is the love the Father has lavished on us, that we should be called children of God! And that is what we are!" 1 John 3:1, NIV.

Can you thank God that He has chosen you as His child? That fact must become real to you. Say it—express thanks to God that you are His chosen one. No matter how you may have been scarred in the past, now, today, your heavenly Father gives you a new identity.

Think of those scarred individuals in the Bible who received a new identity from their Lord. Jacob was known as the cheater, the man who had robbed his own brother of an inheritance. But God gave him a new identity. Jacob became Israel, the father of many nations.

David carried within him the wound of a terrible sin against Bathsheba and Uriah, her husband. But through repentance he found a new identity, as a man after God's own heart.

The thief on the cross bore many scars—his whole life wasted in crime, his heart filled with regret. But a word from the Saviour made him a new man and freed him from the horrible past. Now he was bound for Paradise.

Paul was once haunted by the faces of those he had so zealously persecuted. He had fought against Christ Himself. But one day on the road to Damascus, Jesus gave the persecutor a new identity—Paul, Apostle to the Gentiles.

This same Paul tells us that, as believers, we are "accepted in the Beloved." Ephesians 1:6, NKJV.

Do you recall another time when that word *beloved* was used in Scripture? At Christ's baptism, the Father said, "This is My beloved Son, in whom I am well pleased." Matthew 3:17, NKJV.

How the Father cherished His beloved Son. But listen, that is just how we are cherished. We are accepted in the Beloved. Even as we bare our ugliest scars, even as we reveal those dark, hidden emotions—we are accepted in the Beloved.

When we focus on that truth and claim it for ourselves, we will acquire a Christ-oriented self-image, and true inner healing can begin.

We may have been programmed to belittle ourselves. Our past may have shoved us into a narrow mold—old voices telling us we are not valued, not worth it. But God can reprogram those unhealthy thought patterns.

Listen to the good news of Romans 12:2, NIV: "Do not conform any longer to the pattern of this world, but be transformed by the renewing of your mind."

When you catch yourself falling back into the old pattern, nursing the old wound, accepting that old feeling of worthlessness, *stop*. Claim God's promise to renew your mind. Focus on the new facts. You are chosen as the heavenly Father's child. You are accepted in the Beloved.

Several years ago Corrie ten Boom decided to visit her home town—the quiet little town of Haarlem. Corrie had been away only a few years, but those years—spent in a Nazi concentration camp—seemed like an eternity.

Late one evening she arrived at her old, familiar street. She walked down by the old, familiar houses. In the darkness, she peered through a window into the watchmaker's shop where her father had worked. She ran her hands along the door and listened in the dark.

Corrie remembered the voices of her sister and father and the voices of many friends. All gone now. All victims of the Nazi Holocaust. The walls she stared at were no longer home.

Corrie was left with the horrible memories of a concentration camp. She had seen the worst men can do to each other. She knew many would never recover from the scars left by that experience. Standing alone in the night, Corrie wondered what the future might hold.

Then suddenly a church began to play its familiar chimes. Corrie walked out into the street and paused to look up at the cathedral silhouetted against a black sky and framed by countless twinkling stars.

She remembered the words of Jesus, "Lo, I am with you alway, even unto the end of the world." Matthew 28:20.

Corrie stood there a long time, until the chimes played again. This time "A Mighty Fortress Is Our God" rang out in the night. Yes, Corrie realized, I do have a home in the everlasting arms of my heavenly Father. I have security. And there in the street she thanked the Lord for reminding her of His grace.

Corrie would not be trapped by old scars. Now she was free.

Each of us can be free of the past, each of us can renew our minds, when we truly see that we are accepted in the Beloved. And remember, the Beloved Son is also the Wounded Healer. And He always will be a Wounded Healer.

After Christ's resurrection, He appeared to His disciples in the upper room. Jesus possessed a new, glorified body. He had already appeared in heaven before His Father. And yet this resurrected Lord showed the disciples hands still deeply scarred—and a large wound on His side.

A glorified, risen Saviour—still bearing scars. Why?

Because what happened at Calvary will never be forgotten. I believe that Christ will always bear the scar of the trauma of the cross. The memory of that ordeal will stay with Him throughout eternity.

But the scars are not ugly. In heaven we won't turn our faces away from them. No. They speak of Christ's great sacrifice for mankind. They eloquently symbolize the most beautiful act of love this universe has ever known.

We, too, can't just erase our scars or pretend that they never happened. But God's love can transform them. His grace can fashion a new identity out of old wounds. The past may have been dark, but we can hear His song ringing out in the night. His assurance will come. And we can know that, today, right now, we do have a home in the everlasting arms.

Bribing the Gatekeeper

Many years ago a Chinese emperor built a gigantic wall to defend the country against the barbarians to the north. The wall stretched for miles along the border, and it was wide enough for chariots to pass on its top. It remains one of the wonders of the world. But as a defense effort, the wall was a complete failure. *The enemy breached it by merely bribing a gatekeeper!*

The fiercest, toughest, most decisive battle ever fought is the battle for the mind. It is the mind that decides. It is the mind that chooses. It is the mind that loves. It is the mind that worships. It is the mind that is tempted. The mind is the fortress of the soul. The Creator has built its defenses strong. *But He has made you the gatekeeper.*

What are the weapons in this battle? Words. Billions of words arranged into advertising, crowded into newspapers, bound into books. Words in the air. Words on the screen. Words on the lips of friends or enemies. Words of husbands and wives. Subtle changers of the mind that scar and mold and enslave. Words endlessly repeated. Cutting grooves into the consciousness of willing or unwilling listeners. Shaping characters. And shaping homes.

It was during the Korean War that an American Marine officer, Colonel Frank Schwable, was taken prisoner by the Chinese Communists. And it was not long before it dawned on him that the enemy expected to use him as a tool of propaganda.

The weeks pass. He suffers rough, inhuman treatment, in-

71

timidation, hunger, interrogation for hours on end. He will be better treated, he is told, if he will just unburden himself of guilt. What guilt? he wonders. But soon he finds out. Over the weeks there is a slowly induced hypnosis, and at last, after months of intense psychological pressure, he signs a "confession" that the United States is carrying on germ warfare against the enemy. He gives details.

He said later, "That is the hardest thing I have to explain: how a man can sit down and write something he knows is false, and yet, to sense it, to feel it."

Time, fear, and continual pressure—and never-ending words—had created a menticidal hypnosis. And it could happen to anyone!

A prominent psychiatrist, testifying in the Schwable case, stated that nearly anybody under such circumstances could be forced to sign a similar confession.

"Anyone in this room?" he was asked.

He looked about at the officers sitting in judgment and replied firmly, "Anyone in this room!"

The techniques of brainwashing are becoming more and more precise. The days of witchcraft and torture and the rack may have passed. But the modern refinements of these are here to stay. It is no longer simply a battle for man's body. It is a battle for the mind.

The military aspects, the military possibilities, of such warfare are frightening. Mass brainwashing, mass hypnotism, and drug warfare could subdue whole nations without firing a shot. It is said that a single pound of LSD scattered in the water supply of New York City, with supporting doses, could mentally incapacitate its population long enough for an invading army to take over.

But it is not only the military possibilities that should stagger us. The sweeping hysteria of suggestion is invading the home every day by way of television, radio, and the printed page. We are subjected to a barrage of suggestion, a bombardment of ideas that is slowly conditioning us in areas of life that affect our destiny. And I am not referring to simple advertising.

What we are witnessing is the battle for the mind. More than that, it is the battle for the will of man. And it is a battle for the home.

In every encounter with the forces of evil the battle is fought first, and won or lost, in the mind, before friends or family know it. If ever a man is disloyal to God, to his country, or to his wife, he is disloyal first in the mind. If, as the gatekeeper, he allows temptation free access to the corridors of the mind, there will be no way of escape from the brainwashing forces that will beat against his imagination. And in any conflict between the will and the imagination, usually the imagination wins. Infidelity is the almost inevitable result. It can happen to anyone—anyone who reads this page.

You say, "Pastor Vandeman, do you mean that a man is helpless against temptation? Like Colonel Schwable?"

No. There is one difference. Colonel Schwable was physically forced to remain under the influence of brainwashing propaganda. You are not. You are the gatekeeper. But if you accept the enemy's bribe, if you choose to open your mind to the repetitious rantings of temptation, broken hearts and broken homes are inevitable.

To tamper with the mind is to tamper with the conscience, with the power to decide, with the will. To control the mind is to control the conscience. The mind must be kept strong. It is the unguarded mind that is open to temptation.

The will is the enemy's target. For the will, you see, is the soul's deciding power. It is your decision. It is your choice. Inclination may be strong. Human nature may be weak. But the will decides. The will is the real you.

The will is free. It was never God's will that it should be otherwise. It was never God's plan that any outside influence should control man's will. God *will not* control it without your invitation. Satan *cannot* control it without your permission. It is man who decides.

God never enters the sacred precincts of the conscience uninvited. Satan would like to enter. Family or friends would sometimes like to enter. But God says to the watching universe, "See that man. He is about to make a decision. By that decision he may live or die. But he alone must make it. Stand back! The soul must be free!"

And God Himself waits in the courtyard, stands at the door and knocks, while man decides.

God paid a terrific price to keep the soul free. That price was the death of His Son. It cost the life of Jesus to preserve for you and me the right to choose. God will never force the will. He will only accept it. He wants only willing allegiance.

The enemy, on the other hand, will use any subterfuge, any hellish device to force the will of man.

And so the battle continues. The enemy wants the will of man—to enslave it. God wants the will—to set it free.

What are some of the forces that try to bribe their entry into the mind?

Take hypnotism, for instance. Hypnotism, once regarded as only a harmless parlor game, now comes to us in cap and gown. It professes to free man from undesirable habits. It poses as a great benefactor. But what about the mind? What about the will? When the will is surrendered to another, placed under the control of another, is it not to some extent enslaved and weakened? Is it ever so strong again?

You trust your friend. You trust your counselor. You trust your dentist. But is it ever safe to surrender the will to another? Suppose that in some hypnotic session another intelligence than that of the one you trust should take over. De Witt Miller has put the question this way: "When the subconscious mind, under hypnosis, becomes susceptible to outward suggestions, how can we be sure that some astral interloper of the spirit world will not intrude upon the subconscious mind, in its hypnotic trance-state, and ply its occult arts, as it does with an entranced medium?"—*Reincarnation*, page 37.

It has happened. That is the possibility. That is the danger. Hypnotism is a perilous passkey to the mind. Could it be that hypnotism is delivering on a silver platter what psychic forces have been seeking through the ages—the control of the will?

Is it any wonder that Solomon said, "Keep thy heart [thy mind] with all diligence; for out of it are the issues of life." Proverbs 4:23?

And what of the pills that we swallow by the billions? Are they strengthening the mind, making it more secure against temptation? Or are they subtle bribers at the gate?

Robert S. de Ropp, in his book *Drugs and the Mind*, makes this sparkling comment about our pill-taking generation: "Lucky neurotics! Soon the specter of care will be banished from the world, the burden of anxiety and guilt will be lifted from your souls. The restoration of your primeval innocence, your re-entry into the Garden of Eden, will now be accomplished through the agency of a pill. Soothed by reserpine, calmed by chlorpromazine, mellowed by 'Miltown,' elevated by 'Meratran,' what need you fear from the uncertainties of fortune? Tranquilly, smoothly your days will succeed one another, like the waters of a peaceful river flowing through green pastures in which graze dewy-eyed cows whose state of placid contentment resembles your own. O most fortunate of mortals, whose spiritual defects are made good by the skill of the scientist, whose personal shortcomings are supplemented by a formula. No longer need you struggle with your weaknesses or agonize over your sins. Salvation need not be purchased at the cost of spiritual war. In the chemopsychiatric age you can buy it by the bottle. O brave new world that has such bottles in it!"— Pages 283, 284.

Would you say we are sharpening the sensitivities of the conscience? Making it stronger? Or weakening it pill by pill?

But all this is nothing compared to the psychedelic whirlpool into which this generation is being drawn. The mind-changing drugs, the consciousness-expanding drugs are sweeping the country. Marijuana, LSD, and Methedrine, which makes even LSD pale by comparison.

Every user of LSD is a potential suicide. One boy felt so free that he thought he was God. And so, convinced that nothing could harm him, he walked into oncoming traffic and was almost killed. Users often get delusions of grandeur. They even think they can fly. A boy in Los Angeles was about to throw his girl friend off the roof when the cops caught him. And the worst of it is that you may freak out again, years later, without repeating the drug. I ask you, is it insight? Or is it insanity?

It is estimated that a billion impulses are being sent to our brain every second. Most of them are shut out, fortunately, from our awareness. Someone has suggested that these mind-changing drugs may be dilating the aperture so that more of the impulses get through. This could explain the chaotic nature of the drug experience. At times impulses may be wired directly to the euphoria center, with all other connections unplugged. In that case everything seems fabulously wonderful. But sometimes the connections are not so wired, and the experience is one of nameless horror. In other words, the drug experience may be a temporary rewiring of the brain circuits!

Think of it, friend! Do you see the danger? Do you see what these psychedelic bribers at the gate are doing? Tampering with the mind. Tampering with the seat of decision. Tampering with the conscience. Tampering with a man's eternal destiny!

Is it any wonder that some observers are now speaking of the total annihilation of the will of man?

How jealously we should guard the will! For every influence, every impression allowed entrance to the mind, is shaping the set of the will, determining its future choices and affecting the destiny.

Every time we decide right, we are strengthening the will. And every time we decide wrong, we are weakening the will. It's as simple as that. It may be a little thing, a small decision—as seemingly insignificant as a second piece of pie. But we are either weakening or strengthening the will by that decision. Habits, good or bad, are being strengthened by exercise.

We are wise when we beware of anything that dulls the power of the will. Alcohol can do it. Tobacco can do it. Overeating can do it. Fatigue can do it.

Now someone is saying, "Pastor Vandeman, you're talking about me. I know what I ought to do. But I have absolutely no will power."

That is the cry of thousands of alcoholics. No willpower! And a legion of smokers echo it. No willpower! It is the plaintive cry of millions of weight watchers who put off their weight watching until tomorrow. And the uncounted victims of temper and lust join in. No willpower! It is a cry of defeat that makes the heart of God weep.

I think you can see how intensely practical this is. It is not sufficient to talk to an alcoholic about exercising his will, strengthening his will. For he says hopelessly, "I have none!"

Friend, if we must tie our hopes to our own weakness, or to man-made solutions, or to the manipulations suggested by popular psychology, however helpful their insights, there is reason to despair. For what can a man do when the will is weakened? What can a man do when the will is enslaved by a wrong choice in the past?

Listen. There is hope. For weak though a man may be, he still *has* a will. He still has the *power to choose*. He can *reverse* the unwise decision of the past. He can *choose to change masters*. He can *cry out for deliverance!*

An inspired writer has said it so much better than I can: "The expulsion of sin is the act of the soul itself. True, we have no power to free ourselves from Satan's control; but when we desire to be set free from sin, and in our great need cry out for a power out of and above ourselves, the powers of the soul are imbued with the divine energy of the Holy Spirit, and they obey the dictates of the will in fulfilling the will of God."—*The Desire of Ages*, page 466.

What a paragraph! Read it again and again. Every word of it filled with hope!

Yes, there is hope for the most hopeless. Listen. "Sin shall not have dominion over you." Romans 6:14.

Evidently a man doesn't have to be enslaved by habit. Evidently he doesn't have to see his home disintegrating because of his weakness. Evidently God can break the chains. That's what Jesus came to do.

"The Spirit of the Lord is upon me, because he hath anointed me . . . to preach deliverance to the captives, and recovering of sight to the blind, to set a liberty them that are bruised." Luke 4:18.

Jesus came to break the chains, to set the captive free. He says in John 8:32: "Ye shall know the truth, and the truth shall make you free."

When we learn the truth about what we are discussing here, it will set us free. Not one person who reads this page needs to remain a slave to crippling habit. Every one of you can go free. I say this on the authority of the Word of the living God. "If the Son therefore shall make you free, ye shall be free indeed." John 8:36.

Again, we need to understand that this decisive victory is not achieved by sheer force of self-discipline—by frantic trying. This is made vividly clear in the story of the Indian fakir who once came to a village declaring he would demonstrate how to make gold. The villagers gathered around as he poured water into a huge cauldron, put some coloring matter into it, and began to repeat mantras as he stirred.

When their attention was temporarily diverted, he let some gold nuggets slip down into the water. Stirring a little more, he finally poured off the water, and there was the gold at the bottom of the cauldron.

The villagers' eyes bulged. The moneylender offered 500 rupees for the formula, and the fakir sold it to him.

"But," the fakir explained, "here is the secret. You must not think of the red-faced monkey as you stir. If you do, the gold will never come."

The moneylender promised to remember that he was to forget. But to try to forget is to remember, as the fakir well knew. So try as hard as he might, the red-faced monkey sat on the edge of the moneylender's mind, spoiling all his gold.

Friend, whatever gets your mind gets you. Whatever captures the imagination will enslave you. You can never cast sin out of the mind by trying to forget it. For sin thrives upon attention, even negative attention. Even a loyal attempt to fight sin in the mind can lead to defeat. Do you see now why the sheer force of self-discipline is not enough—why frantic trying doesn't work?

Yes. You cannot control your thoughts and your feelings and your emotions as you may desire. But there is one thing you can do. You can control your will. You can choose who your master shall be. Joshua said, "Choose you this day whom ye will serve." Joshua 24:15.

And that is an act of the will. We choose our master. It will be one—or it will be the other. Every person is under the control of one power or the other—by deliberate choice.

Do you see the constant peril a person is in until he understands the true force of the will? The will is not something to be pushed about by circumstances or smothered under feelings or intimidated by habit or impulse. It need not be subject to the emotions. The life of victory is not to be lived in the emotions, but in the will.

This desire may pull in one direction. This emotion may pull in another. This habit, this temper, this lust may clamor for attention. But the will decides. And the will is the real you.

God does not negotiate with the feelings. He negotiates with the will. In the final destiny of man the feelings are not the deciding factor. It is the will that decides. Let the emotions rebel as they may. They will gradually come into line with the decision of the will. It is yours to decide. And when you do, the power of God, like the lift of the tide, will make all the difference!

I think of the building of a giant bridge across a portion of New York's harbor. Engineers were searching for a base upon which to rest one of the mighty buttresses.

But deep in the mud and practically buried, they discovered an old barge, full of bricks and stones, that had long ago sunk to that spot. It had to be moved. Yet in spite of every device it remained firmly held to its muddy bed.

At last one of the engineers conceived an idea. He gathered other barges about and secured them by long chains to the sunken wreck *while the tide was low*. Then all waited. The tide was coming in. Higher and higher rose the water, and with it the floating barges. Then creaking and straining on the chains, that old boat was lifted from its viselike grip—raised by the lift of the Atlantic Ocean!

Need I draw a parallel?

I ask you, Is your mind like an old barge, full of bricks and stones, gripped by memories you long to forget, held by age-long leanings and habits you would give anything to be released from, bound by fears and uncontrolled imaginations?

Has every human device failed to break the power of their viselike grip in your life? Just know that the lift of the mighty God will deliver you. He is able. But you must choose.

The enemy of God and man is not willing that this priceless secret be clearly understood. For he knows that when you receive it fully, his power will be broken. You will be free—and your home secure!

When the Rain Falls

A young man and his father farmed a small piece of land. Several times a year they would load up a cart with vegetables and take them to market.

The two had little in common. The son was a tense and ambitious individual, the go-getter type. The father, on the other hand, was steady and relaxed.

One morning they loaded the cart, hitched up the ox, and started out for the nearest city. The young man, true to his disposition, kept prodding the ox with a stick. He reasoned that they had a better chance of getting good prices if they reached the marketplace early.

Several hours down the road the father stopped. It was his brother's farm, and he wanted to say hello, for so seldom did he have the opportunity. The son, of course, was impatient at what he considered a needless delay, and did not conceal his restlessness. But the father cautioned, "Take it easy. You'll last longer."

After an hour they drove on. They came to a fork in the road and the father turned to the right. "The other way is shorter," the son reminded him. "Yes, Son. But this way is more beautiful."

"Have you no respect for time?"

"Yes," said the father, "I respect it so much that I like to use it in looking at beautiful things."

At twilight they found themselves in country as lovely as a garden. The father suggested, "Let's sleep here." By this time

81

the boy was angry, and he exploded, "You're more interested in flowers than money!"

But the father quietly replied, "That's the nicest thing you've said in a long time."

"I'll never take a trip with you again!" the boy vowed.

In the morning they were on their way early. Soon they came upon a cart in the ditch, and the father stopped to help while the son, of course, protested. "Take it easy," said the father. "Sometime you might be in the ditch yourself."

And then it was eight o'clock. There was a brilliant flash of lighting. And thunder. "Must be a big rain in the city," said the old man.

"But, Dad, if we had hurried, we could have been sold out by now."

"Take it easy, Son. You'll last longer."

It was late afternoon when they reached the hill overlooking the city. The two men stood for a long moment, looking down. Neither said a word.

And then the son broke the silence. "I see what you mean, Father."

They turned and drove their cart away from what had been, until eight o'clock that morning, *the city of Hiroshima!*

It was not long after the explosion of that first atomic bomb that Bob Ripley originated a broadcast from the ill-fated city. And I heard him say, "I am standing on the spot where the end of the world began!"

Time is running out. We live our days under the ticking of a universal time-fuse. For a generation now we have lived in an atmosphere of tension that is on the verge of hysterics. The tension tolerance of humanity is reaching the breaking point.

We have permitted ourselves to be stampeded into unnatural and dangerous pressures. We hate to miss a single panel of a revolving door. We have compressed our lives into high-speed capsules. We pay with a terrific toll. And it is telling on our homes.

Is there a way to live in this kind of world serenely? How much can we stand? Can these bodies, these minds, these homes take the tensions into which we have been thrust? We live in a broken world. Is it possible to be a whole person in a broken world? Is it possible to relax when the rain falls, and the thunder crashes round our heads? How can we deal with stress in the mind, in the body, in the home?

It was back in 1925 that a young medical student at the University of Prague, burning with enthusiasm for the art of healing, noticed what many physicians before him had noticed, that certain symptoms are common to a great many diseases, and are therefore of little help in making diagnosis. For instance, the fact that a patient feels somewhat ill, has a slight fever, a loss of appetite, and a few scattered aches and pains, would hardly enable a physician to pinpoint the disease.

Young Hans Selye was too new in the medical profession to realize just how laughable his question might sound to his elders—if he should find the courage to ask it. But why, he wondered, had physicians since the dawn of medicine given their attention to understanding the specific symptoms of individual diseases and never troubled themselves to understand the condition of just being sick?

What is it that makes a man sick—not sick with pneumonia or sick with scarlet fever or sick with measles, but just plain sick? Why could not the methods and instruments of research be applied to that problem?

That question in a pioneering young mind was the beginning of a lifetime of research that has resulted in a most valuable contribution to mankind—the better understanding of the stress of life.

Stress, you see, is simply the wear and tear of life. It is what life does to you. Stress is not necessarily caused by some great problem that rolls suddenly upon the mind or body of man. It may be caused by simply crossing a street in traffic, by reading with poor light, by the crying of a baby, by an endless variety of routine everyday occurrences—even by sheer joy.

Now, it is not possible to avoid stress entirely. But it is possible, and very important, to adjust your reaction to it, to strengthen the body's defenses against it. For medical science now knows that many diseases are caused largely by errors in the body's response to stress, rather than by germs or poisons or any other outside agent.

One of Dr. Selye's most valuable, and yet disturbing, contributions has been to point out that every man begins life with a certain reserve of vital force. Once it is gone, it cannot be replaced. It is like a bank account that can be depleted by withdrawals but cannot be increased by deposits.

Many people use up this vitality, restore it from superficial supplies, and are tricked into thinking the loss has been made up by rest. On the contrary, every withdrawal of the deeper reserves of vital force leaves its scar. Somewhere the defenses are wearing thin.

And neither the body nor the mind can take too much wear in the same place. Thousands are in mental hospitals because ruts have been worn in the mind. The same thoughts, the same problems, the same fears and frustrations, have worn a groove deeper and deeper until the mind has become unbalanced. The mind could have stood a variety of problems. But not the same one endlessly repeated.

A man's mind is the most elaborate computer ever devised. But it is too delicate to stand the strain of continuous cutting in the same spot. And overloaded minds, like overloaded electrical circuits, have a way of blowing a fuse. Beyond certain endurance levels the mind and body cannot give.

Do you begin to see what happens in some marital relationships?

Dr. H. S. Liddell and Dr. A. V. Moore, Cornell University psychologists, in experiments upon sheep, disclosed that a series of daily unpleasant incidents, applied with repetition, can in time reduce a sheep to a bleating, neurotic animal and can eventually cause its death.

Let me remind you again of the words of the late Dr. John Schindler: "Most cases of emotionally induced illness are the result of a monotonous drip, drip of . . . unpleasant emotions, the everyday run of anxieties, fears, discouragements and longings."—*How to Live 365 Days a Year*, page 13.

The drip-of-the-faucet experience again. How do you—and I—react to stress that has become familiar by long repetition? That is the question.

Remember the father and son—traveling toward Hiroshima?

In that simple narrative we find some delightful contrasts that help us understand how to deal with stress.

Here were two men, two types, under the same pressures, both traveling toward Hiroshima. They lived in the same world, in the same home, with circumstances they could not change. But their physical, mental, and spiritual reactions were in contrast.

Both were physically fit. Both worked in the open air. But the father had learned how to relax, how to balance work with rest. The son had not.

Their mental attitudes were opposite. Each had a different set of values.

The father trusted his God. The son permitted only selfishness and ambition to rule his life.

Remember the delay as the father visited with his brother? In the son's way of life there was no time for family or friends—only getting ahead. But how many a man has lost his own family, his wife, his children—lost them to self, to society, and to God—because he was too busy!

Remember the cart in trouble? What a contrast between son and father, between selfishness and selflessness! When will we learn the eroding influence of selfishness? When will we learn that sharing is life-giving?

Listen to the words of God through the ancient prophet: "Is not this the fast that I have chosen? to loose the bands of wickedness, to undo the heavy burdens, and to let the oppressed go free, and that ye break every yoke? Is it not to deal thy bread to the hungry, and that thou bring the poor that are cast out to thy house? when thou seest the naked, that thou cover him?" Isaiah 58:6, 7.

And now notice verse 8: "Then shall thy light break forth as the morning, and thine health shall spring forth speedily."

A tremendous promise! A fantastic promise! Many a man, many a woman, has found health when he turned his attention to helping someone else. There is no influence more healing than the spring of unselfishness flowing from within.

And remember the flowers? The father and the son had a different set of values. The father had wisely learned that we are healingly distracted from the tensions of life by the beauties of nature. But the son was a puppet of his stunted philosophy of life.

How much the son missed! And how much we miss of life's richest rewards! We hurl ourselves into life with such reckless abandon that we wring ourselves physically and spiritually dry. We fasten our eyes on some glittering prize of material success. But when we reach it, if we do, we find that the badge of our success is a stomach ulcer or a thrombosis. Stress has taken its toll. The home has suffered. And it didn't need to be that way!

Said Jesus, "Seek ye first the kingdom of God, and his righteousness; and all these things shall be added unto you." Matthew 6:33.

But now one more parallel in our story. The father and son were traveling toward Hiroshima. They didn't know that the bomb would be dropped at eight o'clock that morning. Was it Providence that kept them from being there at that hour? Was it the father's faith? Perhaps so.

But not all who have trusted have been spared. Some have perished when the bombs fell. Some have been burned at the stake. John the Baptist trusted—and was beheaded.

But friend, here is the point. The father's trust did not depend upon God's sparing him from Hiroshima. The father did not know. He only knew his God. He only knew that whatever God permitted was all right with him. Like the patriarch Job he could say confidently, "Though he slay me, yet will I trust in him." Job 13:15.

Are you a victim of tension, anxiety, grasping frustration—like the son? Or is yours a serene, purposeful, selfless confidence—like that of the father? Is your home a picture of tension between father and son, between mother and daughter, or husband and wife? Your home will reflect your own reactions to stress. The way you meet personal stresses and crises and emergencies will be transferred to the family. To keep tension out of the home you must keep it out of the personality.

We may need to remember that, as marriage partners, we can never reach the promised land without going through some wilderness together. And believe me, there will be wilderness. And there will be rain.

It is not necessary to be a practiced diagnostician to see that our world today is not in good health. It is a broken world, a world in deep trouble. War, poverty, and disease are only symptoms. The world is troubled in the spirit.

We are told that every epoch has its own particular malady. The typical sickness of this generation is neurosis. Many doctors agree that more than half their patients suffer from it. And this is not accidental. For our aloof, materialistic, sophisticated society no longer supplies the deeper needs of the soul.

What is neurosis? Simply speaking, a person is neurotic when he represses something without eliminating it. How, then, has neurosis touched this generation? The answer is self-evident. This generation is told so often as to sound convincing that feeling, faith, and Biblical truth are unimportant. Yet men and women at the bottom of their hearts feel a justified intuition that these things are nonetheless important.

Our thirst for love, our spiritual loneliness, our fear of death, the riddle of evil, the mystery of God—we may not speak of these; we may repress them. But they still haunt us. They are repressed but not eliminated. This makes a man sick. This makes a world sick. For in repressing values without having been freed from them, man has repressed the very principle of inner harmony.

What is the result? Modern man, like the adolescent in profound crisis, turns to strange alien behavior. He turns to the bribers at the gate.

Is it possible to be a whole person in a broken world? Is it possible to have a solidly built home, with happiness wall to wall, in a world like this? Even when the rain falls?

It simply must be so. The alternative is to stand one day beside a broken home and view it as a city in shambles, a relationship beyond repair.

One young woman, looking back upon her broken home, realizing where both partners had made mistakes, recalling how they had listened to the unsound counsel of friends, wrote these words:

"The war is over. We stood just now beside the ruins of our

city and used the magic word *forgive*. We understand now. We know now that the city was destroyed by mistake.

"It didn't need to happen. No bomb was dropped upon it. It was carefully built with the best of materials. The voice of prayer was often heard within it. No wonder it had long stood serene and calm against every weapon from without.

"But now it lies in ruins. And we—no one else—we are to blame. You see, we tore it down with words. Your words—my words—words of other people, people who did not understand. But we listened to those words—and began to believe them. And now—

"We were so foolish. We were like children toppling their toy villages. Toppling them with never a care. At first we were afraid. We tried to stop. But one word flamed another until fires broke out in our city that we could not quench. Others were watching now. There were those who liked to see it burn. And then, ignited by hate, our smoldering feelings burst into a final holocaust of words and we abandoned the city.

"We stood beside it just now. The smoking cloud has lifted. Time has cleared our vision. We understand. We forgive. The war is over. But our city is in a shambles. And even forgiveness can never build it again!"

Friend, it need not happen to you or me. Not if we let God teach us the delicate work of mending hearts. Not if we let Him teach us patience and understanding. Not if there is a simple, basic honesty about our own weaknesses—with each other and with God.

Does not the confidence of our mates challenge the best that is in us? I think so. That is why I like the familiar hymn of all churches that says, "I would be true, for there are those who trust me; I would be pure, for there are those who care."

But then it says, "I would be humble, for I know my weakness." Why is such a confession so difficult? It ought not to be. For human nature, whether in friend or marriage partner, will respond dramatically to the honest admission of our own weakness and our own need. Such honesty rules out pretense and sham. It rules out compulsive defending of the personality. Rather, it encourages honest prayer.

Jeanette Struchen has written some "prayers to pray without really trying." But one of them, it seems to me, might take a little courage:

> I need a wrecking crew, Lord.
> I keep building little shabby walls—
>   ego to hide my shortcomings,
>   pride to defend my dishonesty,
>   personal desires to separate me from Your will.
> I put up foundations of prejudice and towers
>   of overconfidence.
> I pile up attitudes into blockades and fortify
>   them with slingshot opinions.
> I erect mighty convictions and brace them up
>   with sand.

I have been reading some of the prayers of the inner city kids, in their own language. Carl Burke has gathered them together.* Here is one that touches a response in any relationship where communication has broken down:

> Dear God—
> Why do religious people
> Always know they
> Are so right
> When they don't give
> Us a chance to talk?

And here is one that is simple, honest, and difficult to say:

> I'm sorry—
> But not sure what that means.
> I'm ashamed—
> But not sure of what.

It makes me think of the words of Paul Tournier: "There is no learned discussion about false or true guilt, but in His grace

---

* Carl F. Burke, *Treat Me Cool, Lord* (New York: Association Press, 1968). Used by permission.

God receives all those who are ashamed." We need not analyze our guilt, or understand it. But we can feel it.

And here is one more prayer from the city streets. Underneath its language you will see a picture of human behavior that is uncannily accurate:

> Lord, we know You s'pose to guide us with Your hand,
> But we don't let You put a finger on us,
> We know You s'pose to guide us with Your eye,
> But we stay outta Your sight;
> That You s'pose to be with us all the time,
> But we make believe You ain't here;
> That You can teach us right from wrong,
> But we ain't listenin' to You,
> Even though You know best.

Sound familiar? Who of us has been so frank to acknowledge our own maneuverings? Does this prayer from the inner city echo your own experience? Does it touch a sensitive response? I confess it does in me.

Why is it that we love each other more when mistakes and weaknesses are admitted? In fact, is a home ever likely to disintegrate while two marriage partners join hands before an understanding God and face their problems honestly? Hardly!

There will be stress. There will be rain. And there may have been disloyalty. But God has not been caught unprepared. Long before science taught us that we had a subconscious mind to contend with, with inherited tendencies to selfishness, with filth that rises to rest like scum upon the surface of the mind—I say, before we ever learned these terms, the Word of God showed us how even these deepest areas could be cleansed and changed.

Thank God, we don't need to accept ourselves as we are. Conversion is possible even for the subconscious mind. When a man consents to the healing stroke of Omnipotence, when a man invites the divine invasion of his soul, he can know that that touch of purity will sink to the depths and cleanse and sweeten and purify. It will leave him clean. And it will leave him kind!

What would you give for a cleansing like that? What would such a change do for your home? What would such a possibility mean to those you love? You've promised them the best. Heaven will help you give it!

Papa, Are You Going to Die?

An old legend tells of a Portuguese monastery that stood precariously atop a three-hundred-foot cliff. Visitors were strapped in a huge wicker basket and then pulled to the top with an old ragged rope. As one visitor stepped into the basket for the descent, he asked anxiously, "How often do you get a new rope?"

"Whenever the old one breaks," a monk calmly replied.

Risky. Dangerous. Like hurtling through life on a threadbare rope—ready to break!

Skidding along! Getting by! Getting by with the aid of too many cups of coffee, too many cigarettes, too much wound-up nervous energy—and too little sleep, relaxation, fun and frolic. Spending five dollars' worth of energy on a five-cent problem. Tense, parchment-faced individuals who cannot decide whether to take a Benzedrine and go to a party or take a Seconal and go to bed!

In this hurry-scurry, pell-mell, atomic age of jets, speed, and spasm we take too little time to live sanely. We career down the highway of modern life until our health is gone. And then, with our time and with our money, we pay. Too late we discover that when the rope breaks, it cannot be replaced. The Creator gave us only one!

Now everybody knows, of course, that someday the rope will break. It does—sometime—for every man. But the question is this: *Does it have to break so soon?*

A recent book on airline safety—or lack of it—is entitled *It*

Doesn't Matter Where You Sit. I got the impression that the author feels there are so many possibilities for disaster in the air that a safe arrival may be largely a matter of luck. He debunks the idea that riding in the tail section is safer. Despite his scholarly presentation of the facts of airline safety, pro and con, his thinking seems to be at least somewhat influenced by the fatalistic idea that when your number comes up, the plane will crash.

Unfortunately, many people extend that fatalistic philosophy to every area of life—not just to air travel. It doesn't matter where you sit. It doesn't matter how you live. It doesn't matter how you eat—or drink—or smoke. There's nothing you can do about it anyway. When the rope is suppose to break—according to some fatalistic computer—it will break. So just live as you please—until your number rolls around.

Now I don't believe in this number business. I do believe in a divine Providence. My Bible tells me that not a sparrow falls to the ground without God's awareness—certainly much less an airline passenger. But I don't subscribe to blaming some mystical number when a man drives his car off a cliff while under the influence of alcohol—or to blaming the will of God when a man has dug his own grave with his teeth.

Tell me. If some elusive but all-powerful number is in control, why is it that smokers live shorter lives than other men? Why is it that life-insurance companies consider an overweight individual a high risk? Why do those who exercise have fewer heart attacks, and therefore live longer? Does it just happen?

Ancient Israel suddenly becomes both interesting and relevant now that we have all become ecology-minded. For did you know that in ancient Israel God provided for the nations a pattern, a pilot program that, if followed in principle today, would do much to solve the problems of our environment?

You are probably aware that God gave the Israelites a variety of laws, rules, and regulations on their way from Egypt to Palestine. You may have thought that all of these laws were religious in nature, having to do only with moral issues, or at least extending only to ceremony and ritual. This is not true.

Many of Israel's laws, given by God Himself, were given to them for the protection of their environment.

Here they were, six hundred thousand men, beside women and children—with the hygienic background of slaves—traveling through a hot desert without conveniences or medical supplies. What a perfect setting for an epidemic! Yet it didn't happen. Or perhaps I should qualify it by saying that the only recorded epidemics on this long journey were the result of direct disregard of divine instruction.

True, they were in the open air. But every precaution was taken against the pollution of that air. No human waste of any kind was allowed within the encampment, and all possible control was exerted in its proper care elsewhere. See Deuteronomy 23:12-14. This concern for cleanliness was each person's first line of defense against sickness and the community's protection against pollution and pestilence. The well-being of each person depended on how carefully every other person cared for human waste and the delicate balances in nature.

All who were in contact with contaminating diseases were isolated from the camp, were quarantined until they and every person they had touched, and every thing they had touched, were cleansed and declared safe. See Leviticus 15:4-12. And later, in the towns they inhabited, if a house was declared unfit for human habitation, it was destroyed before the pollutions resulting from decay could set in. See Leviticus 14:45, 47.

Now if you think the understanding of ecology and sanitation given to Israel was simply a reflection of the accepted medical thinking of the time, you are mistaken. Somewhere around the year 1552 B.C., not long before Moses was born in Egypt, a famous Egyptian medical book was written. It is called *Papyrus Ebers* and no doubt accurately reflects the medical knowledge of that day. Would you like to hear two or three of the prescriptions from that book?

"To prevent the hair from turning gray, anoint it with the blood of a black calf which has been boiled in oil, or with the fat of a rattlesnake."

For falling hair this was prescribed: "When it falls out, one remedy is to apply a mixture of six fats, namely those of the horse, the hippopotamus, the crocodile, the cat, the snake, and the ibex. To strengthen it, anoint with the tooth of a donkey crushed in honey."

Victims of the bite of poisonous snakes, in that day, received from physicians a "magic water" to drink—water that had been poured over a special idol. And to embedded splinters they applied worms' blood and asses' dung. Since dung is loaded with tetanus spores, is it any wonder that lockjaw took a heavy toll of splinter cases?

Undoubtedly Moses, with his preparation for the royal court, was familiar with *Papyrus Ebers*, and his people with its remedies. It was to this people that God gave the completely revolutionary principles of ecology and hygiene that were millenniums ahead of their time.

It did, in fact, take science thousands of years to catch up. For instance, a disease then thought to be leprosy—medical authorities now believe it probably was syphilis—killed countless millions during the Middle Ages. And what finally brought it under control? The physicians had nothing to offer. Some of them thought it was brought on by eating hot food, pepper, and garlic. Others believed it to be caused by malign conjunction of the planets. It was the church that took a hand. The church went back to the book of Leviticus to discover how to deal with contagion. Taking their cue from Moses, they segregated the patients, excluded them from the community, and the disease was brought under control.

Then there was the Black Death, a killer that took the lives of an estimated seventy-five million in medieval times. The same Biblical concepts of dealing with contagion were applied to the Black Death, and it too was finally controlled.

It was in the 1840s, a little more than a century ago, that a young doctor by the name of Ignaz Semmelweis was given charge of an obstetrical ward in one of the famous teaching hospitals of Vienna, a medical center of that day. Dr. S. J. McMillen, in his book *None of These Diseases*, recounts the tragic story.

Women who died were wheeled into the morgue for autopsy. Every morning, physicians and medical students came into the morgue and performed the autopsies. And then, *without washing their hands*, the doctors with their retinue of students marched into the maternity wards to make pelvic examinations of the living women—of course with no rubber gloves. One out of every six patients died.

Dr. Semmelweis noticed that it was particularly the women examined by these teachers and students who died. After watching this heartbreaking situation for three years, he made a rule that, in his ward, doctors and students coming from the autopsies must wash their hands.

In April, 1847, before this rule was put into effect, fifty-seven women had died in his ward. In June, after the rule, only one in forty-two women died; in July, one in eighty-four.

But one day, after performing autopsies and washing their hands, the doctors and students examined twelve women in a row without washing after each examination. Eleven of the twelve quickly developed high temperatures and died. Evidently fatal infection had been carried from one patient to the others. So the new rule was that hands must be washed following each examination.

Was Dr. Semmelweis acclaimed by his fellows for this breathtaking breakthrough? No. Hand-washing was a nuisance. Prejudice forced him to leave the hospital. His successor threw out the wash basins, and the mortality rates shot back up to the old figures.

Heartbroken, he went to Budapest and once again brought down the death rates. But his colleagues would not speak to him in the hospital corridors. His sensitive nature was so crushed by the prejudice of his fellows, and so haunted by the death cries of dying mothers, that his mind finally broke. He died in a mental hospital without ever receiving the recognition he so richly deserved.

Yet thousands of years before, God had given Moses detailed instructions about cleansing the hands after handling the dead or the infected living!

Yes, the laws of ancient Israel, given by God Himself, and so out of step with the primitive medical knowledge of that day, were far ahead of their time. And it was to this people, fresh out of slavery, long subject to the diseases of the Egyptians, and well aware of the uselessness of the accepted remedies—it was to this people that God made a fantastic promise:

"If thou wilt diligently hearken to the voice of the Lord thy God, and wilt do that which is right in his sight, and wilt give ear to his commandments, and keep all his statutes, I will put *none of these diseases* upon thee, which I have brought upon the Egyptians: for I am the Lord that healeth thee." Exodus 15:26.

Think of it! None of these diseases. And as long as Israel carried out its part of the bargain, God carried out His. Says David, "There was not one feeble person among their tribes." Psalm 105:37.

Now I ask you, Was this remarkable freedom from disease just a miracle? Was it simply an arbitrary reward? Or were the Israelites so free from disease at least partly because of their meticulous attention to their environment?

Evidently there is something we can do about disease and death. Maybe it is not some mystical number that controls our fate. Maybe it is not the stars. Maybe it does matter where we sit—if we sit too long at the dinner table, or lounge too long in our favorite chair when we ought to be out jogging or planting a garden or building a boat!

Jim Hampton's four-year-old daughter had been watching television. And then she looked him straight in the eye and asked him, "Papa, are you going to die?"

Four-year-old girls can be so innocent and disarming and irresistible with their questions. I know.

Jim Hampton was thrown a little off balance by his daughter's words. Not because he didn't know that every father has to be prepared to explain death to his children. Difficult as it always is, he was ready for that. He could explain, as well as any parent, that death eventually comes to every person. It is one of the facts of life—never understood, perhaps, but accepted nonetheless.

But this was different. You see, that was not all she said. There were two more words. What she really said was, "Papa, are you going to die *from smoking?*"

That was different. That was embarrassing. That was something he ought to be able to do something about. He could blame death to the facts of life—but not death from smoking. He—not fate, not some evil entity, not the divine will—he was the problem. That's why Jim Hampton kicked the habit.

Other four-year-olds, in other circumstances, might ask the equally embarrassing question, "Are you going to die from overweight?" Or when they get a little older, they might silently wonder, "Are you going to die from stress?" "Are you going to die from inactivity?"

And so—the book that you hold in your hand is not a book about death. It is not a book about what happens to a man when he dies. Rather, it is intended to help you postpone the day when the rope breaks, the day when your wife becomes a widow, or your husband a widower.

And in the meantime—I promise you—life can be more exciting, more meaningful, and more fun!

How to Burn Your Candle

Nine-year-old Tommy, wet and bedraggled in his angel costume and yellow wig, sat in a tree not far from the bridge that might collapse at any moment. He had been at the school, practicing for the Easter pageant. He hadn't wanted to go. After all, what nine-year-old boy wants to be cast as an angel with wings and yellow curls? But his mother had insisted.

On the way home a violent storm had come up. Tommy knew that the bridge could not be trusted in a storm. It was one that a group of neighbors had built to save going ten miles around the lake. His father had told him, in a situation like this, just to climb a tree and wait for him to come after him. So Tommy was waiting.

Through the dense fog he saw lights approaching. As the car came into view, he saw that it was old Sandy McPherson. None of the neighbors had ever seen Sandy sober. If he had been drinking now, and he almost certainly had, he might not use good judgment. He might drive onto the precarious bridge.

So Tommy called out as loud as he could, "Sandy, don't take the bridge! Go around the lake!"

Tommy started to climb down, for surely Sandy would take him home. But Sandy took off as if he had seen a ghost!

A few minutes later Tommy's father, on his way to pick up his boy, met Sandy on the road. Sandy got out of his car—pale, his lips quivering, his hands shaking. For the first time in anyone's memory, he was cold sober. "You won't believe me," he gasped, "but I just saw a vision! God hasn't forgotten me! The good God—He hasn't forgotten!"

His friend tried to calm him. "Take a deep breath and tell me slowly. You must get hold of yourself."

"Well, I'd had a few drops of whiskey, to keep the chill off, you understand. It was getting dark and the visibility was zero. I was about to turn onto the bridge when I heard a voice say, "Sandy, don't take the bridge! Go around the lake!"

Sandy continued, still out of breath. "I looked up, and there, floating between the trees, was an angel! Dressed in white he was, with wings on his shoulders, and yellow curls on his head!"

"What did you do?"

"I threw my bottle out with all my force. If the good God thinks enough of old Sandy McPherson to send an angel to warn him, I won't be a party to destroying myself!"

And Sandy was never known to take another drink!

Sandy McPherson's candle was almost burned out when he made that important decision. But millions haven't made it yet. No angel in yellow curls has come to warn them. And they've been too busy burning their candle—recklessly at times—to notice the erratic flickering of the flame!

There is something intriguing about lifting a new candle from its wrapping. Its pristine freshness, its unscarred form, and its delicate decoration seem to invite us never to burn it at all. At least they call forth resolutions of carefulness.

But candles are for burning. Life is for living. The wick must be blackened if there is to be light. How we burn it is the theme of this chapter and several that follow—and a matter we neglect at our peril. Either we use the flame with care—or we become a statistic. The choice is ours!

Life is a parade of people. People going somewhere or coming back, pursuing something or waiting for something to pursue them. It's a parade that surges with the rush hour, slowing in the heat of the day. People, each in his own way, burning the candle—and never giving it a thought until its malfunctioning heartbeat warns that time is short!

They've been such good procrastinators. Always waiting for tomorrow. Taking better care of their cars than their bodies. As if they could turn them in on a new model just any time!

Besides, reason millions, when your number comes up, that's

it! There's nothing you can do about it!

The Pasadena Community Church, in St. Petersburg, Florida, was surrounded by pine trees. But in one season two of them were struck and damaged by lightning and had to be cut down. At a meeting of the official board all present were bemoaning the loss of their trees and wondering what could be done to prevent further destruction. Someone asked the chairman, "What can we do? We can't keep losing our trees!"

The chairman replied, with tongue in cheek, "I shall entertain a motion by this body to have the lightning stopped!"

Unfortunately, lightning is one of a number of things that are not subject to committee action!

And many people seem to think our health, and how long we live, are like the lightning—something we can't do anything about. When our number comes up, when the lightning strikes, we're finished. Nothing we can do about it. So why worry?

Now I will agree that we can't control the lightning. Neither can we take a committee vote and stop all illness and all aging and all death. Oh that we could!

But do we have to invite tragedy by standing near a tree in a thunderstorm? And do we have to invite the breakdown of health by the reckless way we burn our candles? Have we forgotten that there is such a thing as the law of cause and effect?

A very little girl said to a friend over thirty, "Your face is all wrinkled." And the friend responded, "Well, how do you suppose it got wrinkled?"

The little girl was wiser than she knew when she said thoughtfully, "Somebody wrinkled it."

Our wrinkles and our ulcers and our heart attacks don't just happen. They are the result of stress somewhere—within or without the body. Somebody or something did it. We live in an age of stress and anxiety and tension. And it tells in our faces— and in our arteries, and on our nerves!

It is said that in the year 1895 there were only two automobiles in the entire state of Ohio. And what happened? You guessed it. They collided!

Cars have been colliding ever since—in constantly increasing numbers. And we've learned to go farther and faster.

Planes have been getting bigger and noisier. Even the air lanes are congested. Our neighbors are no longer five miles away. They're five feet away. We can't seem to catch up with life. We get more and more involved. The pace of life accelerates. We're caught in a revolving door!

And what happens? We burn our candles too fast!

Let me repeat. Dr. Hans Selye, the world's leading authority on stress, has pointed out that every man begins life with a certain reserve of vital force. Once it is gone, it cannot be replaced. Many people use up this vitality and then try to restore it with a few hours or a few days of rest. But it doesn't work that way. Every withdrawal of these deeper reserves of vital force leaves its scar. We have only so much candle!

Now stress is not all bad. It's what keeps our hearts beating and our lungs breathing while we sleep. "Complete freedom from stress is death," says Dr. Selye.

It's too much stress that gives us problems—too much and all the time. Our bodies are perfectly equipped for the amount of tension we were intended to experience.

The body, under sudden stress, reacts quickly and dramatically. The heart beats faster. Vision and hearing improve. The lungs take in more oxygen. The muscles are able to do what they can't do at any other time.

This response is fine, it is adequate, for shoveling snow or cutting down a tree. It is just what you need for jumping out of the way of a speeding car or if a bear is chasing you. But you can't cut down trees nonstop. And if a bear is chasing you all the time, you're in trouble!

The body was never meant to be constantly in a state of alert. And the problem is that physical danger, physical exertion, is not the only thing that triggers the body's reaction. Most of us aren't chased by a bear very often. Some of us haven't had to cut down a tree yet. But the body's fight-or-flight response is also triggered by an unkind word from the boss, an argument with a friend, a feeling of being unappreciated, a stunning defeat—or even a stunning victory. These may have the same consequences as a threat to our physical safety. The body doesn't know that we aren't chopping down a forest!

What does stress do to us? It gives us ulcers, heart attacks, high blood pressure, migraine headaches, and mental illness. It lowers our resistance to disease. It has a lot to do with aging. There is some evidence that it may even trigger certain cancers. In other words, stress can take years off our lives!

"Stress," according to Dr. Selye, "is unquestionably the major health problem in the world today." He says, "It's a killer!"

Stress can be lethal. But let me emphasize again that stress is not all bad. Nor does it originate only in unpleasant experiences. It is easy to understand that stress results from the loss of a loved one—or from losing one's job. But it is also present when you take a vacation or move into a new home or redecorate the old one. Stress is simply the wear and tear of life!

The big problem, then, is not the presence of stress. The problem is how you react to it, what you do with it!

NBC's Dr. Art Ulane, speaking of tension headaches, says that they are caused by literally wearing our scalps too tight. He says we react to stress by clenching our fists, setting the jaw, and tightening the muscles of the scalp.

In other words, we fight back. And it's the fighting back that gives us trouble!

Dr. Claire Weekes, an Australian physician, has had remarkable success in treating people who suffer overwhelming anxiety at the thought of traveling alone, leaving the safety of their homes, or being "caught" in crowded places. She discovered that what these people really fear is the panic they experience in these situations. They fear the *symptoms* of their anxiety.

And how does Dr. Weekes treat these people? By teaching them four concepts, four attitudes toward their problem: "facing, accepting, floating, letting time pass." Or in slightly more detail: "face—do not run away; accept—do not fight; float—do not tense; let time pass—do not be impatient with time."

And it works! Dr. Weekes says it will work equally well for victims of general anxiety—not just those who have the problems mentioned. She says, "Floating is the opposite of fighting. I have occasionally cured a patient in an anxiety state by using the simple words, 'Float. Don't fight!'"

But you know how it goes. We tense when we are behind

schedule—when we have too much to do and not enough time. We tense when a driver honks his horn at us, or cuts in ahead of us. We tense when some member of the family is in a bad mood. We tense when somebody keeps us waiting. We tense when we spend hours shopping and don't find a thing we were looking for. We tense when somebody says an unkind word to us. We tense when we are blamed for something we didn't do.

Tension. Worry. Anxiety. Panic. All these add up to stress. And stress, sooner or later, means illness!

If only we could learn to take the wear and tear of life in stride—and not let it disturb us!

Sidney Harris, writing in the Chicago *Daily News* some years ago, told of walking to the newsstand with a Quaker friend. The friend bought a paper and thanked the newsboy politely. The boy only grunted.

"A solemn fellow, isn't he?" Mr. Harris commented.

"Yes, he's that way every night."

"Yet I noticed that you went out of your way to be courteous to him."

And the Quaker friend replied, *"Why should I let him decide how I am going to act?"*

Is it possible that the answer to stress is simpler than we have thought?

Is it possible that if the candle of life were to come to us complete with printed instructions, like many things we buy in the stores—is it possible those instructions might read something like this? "For best results get plenty of sunlight. An abundance of water, used outside and in, will do wonders. Adequate rest is important. Fresh air, outdoors and indoors, is absolutely essential. The value of exercise cannot be overemphasized. A healthful diet is a must. And trust in God will do more for your candle than anything else."

And then there might be a warranty with our candle—a warranty including these words: "With care, your candle will give you many years of enjoyment. But the Creator is not responsible for damage or loss caused by neglect or misuse."

Burn your candle carefully, friend. There is only one to a customer!

Exercise— Toy or Tool?

Dr. Kenneth Cooper, of *Aerobics* fame, tells of a young man who had had a series of what he was told were heart attacks. He became so depressed that he decided to end his life. But he wanted to do it in some way that would not be recognized as suicide.

So one evening he kissed his wife and his children goodbye and left the house. He ran as fast and as hard as he could until he fell from exhaustion. For a man who had had several heart attacks that certainly should do the trick. But much to his surprise, he didn't die. So he crawled home.

The next evening he did the same thing. But again he survived.

At the end of the first week he noticed that he was running farther and faster. After four weeks he could run for thirty minutes and return home at a brisk trot. And at the end of six weeks he was so strong and happy that he decided to go on living.

Now it is evident that what had been described as heart attacks were not heart attacks at all. But even with a perfectly healthy heart he was doing a very dangerous thing that none of you should try. It is never safe for anyone not used to exercise to plunge suddenly into a vigorous exercise program.

But here is the point. Exercise, in this case running, cured his depression. Doctors say they are not quite sure why this is so, although again and again it has been demonstrated that exercise does relieve depression.

Persons with a life history of migraine headaches have reported that their headaches stopped after a few weeks of physical training. And one study has shown that a vigorous fifteen-minute walk reduces neuromuscular tension more effectively than 400 milligrams of a tranquilizer. In other words, exercise helps you relax. And unquestionably exercise produces favorable changes in the brain.

Better put on your most comfortable walking shoes and be on your way. Because if you don't keep fit, you're in trouble!

We are told that Nicolo Paganini, the great composer and violinist of the nineteenth century, willed his violin to the Italian town where he was born. But there was one condition. No one should ever play this wonderful instrument again.

The violin was placed on exhibition under a glass case in the city hall. Many years passed, and the stipulation that it should not be played was forgotten. A famous violinist came to town for a concert and wanted to try the great Paganini's instrument. He was given permission. But when the violin was picked up, it fell apart. The worms had been eating it as it lay there unused.

A violin is made to be used. So are the muscles of our body. Disuse can have drastic consequences.

Children usually have no trouble getting enough exercise. From the time they are born they seem to be constantly in motion. Exercise comes naturally. It isn't a chore they have to perform. It isn't a tool to achieve physical fitness. To children it's a toy. It's fun!

The old swimming hole of years past may have been replaced by the heated pool in the backyard. But it's still fun. It's recreation. It isn't something kids do to get an increase in their weekly allowance.

Teenagers who live near the ocean aren't fulfilling some dream of Mom and Dad when they are out there surfboarding. They're out there every chance they get. This is life! This is what it's all about!

And when they take off to the mountains in the winter for a weekend on the ski slopes they probably aren't training for the Olympics. This is living! And they could take a lot more of it if only there were more snow on the slopes the year round.

But a lot of teenagers don't live near the ocean or near the snow. So they do with what they have, which is concrete. There's a concrete ribbon from coast to coast. And the skateboarders are riding it. It may be a dangerous sport. Yet statistically it is much safer than riding a bicycle or taking a bath!

Dangerous or not, the kids are keeping fit and calling it fun. It's too bad this ever changes. But it does. Somewhere along the road to maturity exercise, for many people, ceases to be a toy and becomes a tool. And the tool is put away in its kit, to be taken out and dusted off less and less frequently.

And we are paying the price!

The sad thing is that when the bill comes due and somebody we know pays for his inactive life with a heart attack, we call it an act of God. Somebody pays for his own neglect, and we say God did it. Somebody dies from overeating, and we say it was the will of God. Somebody drinks and drives and collides with a telephone pole, or worse with a carload of innocent people; and we wonder why God permits such a tragedy.

What do we expect Him to do? Suspend the law of gravity, the laws of motion, the laws of physics, and the simple laws of health—so that we can violate them at will?

Forgive me for mentioning lifestyle again. But did you know that the five leading causes of death in men thirty-five to fifty-four years of age in the United States are all related to our lifestyle? Here they are. The first is heart disease, which evidence indicates can be prevented, or at least delayed, by adequate exercise, a proper diet, watching our weight, and avoiding tobacco.

Then comes lung cancer, which we all know is directly related, in most cases, to the use of tobacco.

The third leading cause of death is auto accidents. And alcohol is too often the culprit.

Fourth is cirrhosis of the liver. Again alcohol is the prime suspect.

And the fifth leading cause of death is strokes. The most common cause of strokes is high blood pressure. And overeating, overweight, is frequently the cause of high blood pressure.

Now I ask you, How many of these five leading causes of death are acts of God, and how many are acts of men?

The apostle Paul gave us some good counsel when he said, "So whether you eat or drink or whatever you do, do it all for the glory of God." 1 Corinthians 10:31, NIV.

Is it for the glory of God that we permit our bodies, our lives, to be sacrificed to our neglect?

Paul makes it still plainer in these words: "Do you not know that your body is a temple of the Holy Spirit, who is in you, whom you have received from God? You are not you own; you were bought at a price. Therefore honor God with your body." 1 Corinthians 6:19, 20, NIV.

Are we honoring God with our bodies? Are we honoring God with our inactivity, with our overrich and overstimulating diet, with our lazy habits, with our addiction to a weed? Are we treating our bodies as we would a temple? Or do we sometimes treat them as if they were trash cans? Are we as careful with our bodies as we are with our cars?

Paul says, "If anyone destroys God's temple, God will destroy him; for God's temple is sacred, and you are that temple." 1 Corinthians 3:17, NIV.

But does this mean that God will arbitrarily punish us if we destroy our bodies—as a sort of revenge? Or does it mean that God, because He does not force the will, will stand by and *permit* us to destroy our own bodies if that is what we insist on doing?

Listen. Our Lord wants to save the whole man, including his body. But we don't give Him a chance. So often we get in the way of what He wants to do for us. Our resolutions are so good. And our performance is so bad. We seem to be locked into a lifestyle that doesn't work any wonders for our health.

Baseball, for instance, is great exercise for those who play it. But it doesn't do much for those who merely watch—and snack!

For too long we've just gone our way, seldom thinking of our health until something hits us. And then it may be too late to do anything about it.

For instance, do you realize that very often the first symptom of heart disease is sudden death? And what can we do about it then? Heart disease may be developing for twenty years. But it may take only seconds to kill us. We need to do something about those twenty years!

Stress is definitely a factor in heart disease. And exercise controls stress. Dr. Hans Selye, whom we have mentioned before as the world's leading authority on stress, demonstrated this in an experiment with two groups of mice. One group was kept in a cage for a month without any facilities for exercise. Then they were exposed to a variety of unpleasant conditions—electrical impulses, unusual noise, flickering lights. The mice couldn't take it. They all died in a short time.

Mice in the other group were forced to exercise in the cage for several hours each day. When they were exposed to the same unpleasant conditions, they were unaffected. They played, did exercises with the spinning wheel, ate well, got their sleep, and lived on with no sign of a problem.

Doesn't this suggest how much we need exercise—if we expect to cope with everyday stress? Evidently if we don't use exercise as a toy, then we'd better use it as a tool!

What kind of exercise? That's the question.

Jogging has achieved great popularity in the past few years. Millions of people jog. And many people run—particularly athletes. But running is too vigorous for the majority of people. And there is evidence that jogging is not as safe as we once thought. It should not be attempted except on the advice of your physician. And even then there may be a question.

There have been a number of instances, unfortunately, in which people have had a heart attack and died while jogging. Defenders of jogging, of course, will tell you that people die when they're doing other things too. People die in their sleep, and we don't stop sleeping because of that. The argument seems sound enough. And yet why not be safe? It is always possible that the condition of your heart is not apparent to your physician, that developing heart disease is there but has not shown up in any examination. And there is always danger, I say again, when vigorous exercise is attempted by one who is not accustomed to it.

My own experience with jogging has been a happy one. In my book *Papa, Are You Going to Die?* I have related how I started to jog after a frightening health crisis. I jogged for many years, but now I am walking—walking several miles a day. And now I've added tennis!

But my words of caution still stand.

One further word on walking. It may take a little more time to get the amount of exercise you need. But there is no better exercise than walking. And there are no counts against it. Dr. Kenneth Cooper, certainly an expert in the field, says that walking is safe even for a person with undiagnosed heart disease.

Walking forces you to take in more oxygen. It requires no equipment. It's pleasant. You can enjoy it.

But there's something special about walking—something especially good. In the veins of the legs a series of valves open and close while you walk. As the muscles contract with each step you take, the blood is forced upward toward the heart. Then in between steps the valves close. So as you walk, the valves alternately open and close. In this way the leg muscles force the blood up the leg toward the heart, taking some of the work load off the heart. Your legs act as a sort of second pump!

I think you can see that walking greatly improves the circulation of the blood. And I wonder if you realize just how important that is. Many people are invalids simply because the blood does not circulate freely. Processes necessary to life and health do not take place. Exercise, by promoting the circulation, would remedy the situation. But there are people who refuse to exercise—and actually die for the want of it!

Circulating blood, you see, must carry both oxygen and nutrients to every cell of the body. Anything that reduces the flow of blood reduces well-being. As circulation fails, energy fails. In other words, our health, our well-being, our nutrition, our energy, our endurance all depend upon the fitness of the circulatory system. And exercise is the way to keep the circulating blood fit and performing as it was meant to perform.

Walking, then, is good for the heart. It improves the circulation and delivers more oxygen to the cells. It gives you more energy. It relieves tension. It promotes sleep. It fights aging. No pills. No expensive equipment. Just your own two feet—and the will to get started.

Walking is not the only good exercise, of course. Swimming is good. Cycling is good. Winter sports and water sports. There is plenty of variety if you just look for it. Even singing while you work will give you an extra intake of oxygen. And oxygen is the key.

If possible, find an exercise you can enjoy. Make exercise a toy, a recreation, if you can. But if you can't, then make it a tool and exercise anyway!

Somebody reading these words will add years to his life. It could well be you!

The Menu and the Mind

Could it be—is it possible—that innocent-looking menus can tamper with the mind?

A young woman stepped into a doctor's office and was seated. She looked exhausted.

"I can hardly get any real sleep," she began. "Last night it was a little better. I only got up to iron my sheets five times."

The doctor wondered if he had heard correctly. "Did you say you got up to iron your sheets five times?"

"Yes, that's what I said."

She went on to explain. It seems that she simply couldn't stand the slightest wrinkle. If she felt one, she couldn't go to sleep. She had to get out of bed and iron her sheets. She had done this as many as twenty-five times in a single night. But last night hadn't been so bad. It was only five times!

As the doctor talked with her, he soon discovered the trouble. She was evidently a very hungry person. But she was living on nothing but bread and milk twice a day. Her food intake was at the near-starvation level. Why?

"Dad kicks on the grocery bill," she said, "so I don't eat much." And she added that she didn't know why he was so stingy, because he had property all over town.

After six months on an adequate diet she was able to sleep through almost every night without getting up to iron her sheets.

Now please don't anybody say that George Vandeman said if you don't eat right, you'll have to get up at night to iron your sheets! The story I have just told you is true. But it's an extreme instance of what can happen. Undoubtedly it won't happen to you or anybody you know.

On the other hand I can't promise that you won't experience something worse if you aren't careful how you eat. For I'm sure you will agree that there are a lot of things worse than ironing sheets at night—even though they don't make as good a story!

I could tell you other instances almost as spectacular. There was the wife of a young attorney, happily married. Suddenly one night, without warning, she rushed over to the fireplace, took one of her husband's golf trophies from the mantel, and threw it through the window. She ran screaming from the house and didn't come back for three hours. The next day she asked her husband how the window got broken!

She had been on a reducing diet.

There was a young man who was suffering from severe claustrophobia—fear of small enclosures. Believe it or not, he had been unable to take a bath or a shower for over five years. He simply couldn't stay in the bathroom long enough to shower without being overcome by sheer panic!

He had been eating nothing but hamburger. He did say he "balanced" it with coffee and skim milk. And he smoked cigarettes incessantly.

There was the eighteen-year-old girl who described herself as a mental case. She was afraid of glass doors and big glass windows, stairways, elevators, bridges, tunnels, traffic, and germs.

Her diet was practically all refined carbohydrate foods. She recovered in a few weeks after changing her eating pattern.

Again, these are extreme cases. I'm not suggesting that you won't be able to take a shower if you eat hamburger! Or that you will start throwing things through the window if you try to reduce! Or that you will be afraid of everything from elevators to germs if your diet isn't perfectly balanced!

Nevertheless, it is common knowledge in medical and nutritional circles that diet does influence behavior. And sometimes it makes people do some pretty strange things.

Some years ago the University of Minnesota conducted an interesting study. Thirty male volunteers, all of them psychologically normal, were placed on a near-starvation diet for six months. And what happened? The group as a whole showed marked personality changes, both neurotic and psychotic. Some became so disturbed that they even inflicted physical damage on themselves.

So it is not only what you eat, but what you don't eat, that can give you trouble. There is plenty of documentation that mental disturbances and damage to the nervous system can result from a diet deficient in certain vitamins.

Dr. U. D. Register, Loma Linda University nutritionist, says that "in a thiamine or vitamin B^1 deficiency a person becomes irritable, depressed, quarrelsome, uncooperative, fearful of impending misfortune, forgetful, and apathetic. He feels uneasy, has ideas of persecution, disturbing dreams, vague fears, and delusions."

He says that in a niacin (a B vitamin) deficiency "a person may be depressed, emotionally unstable, irritable, fearful, confused, disoriented, and delirious, and may have hallucinations and be stuporous."

I am not suggesting that *all* emotional problems have their origin in the type of diet we choose, or that is available to us. But I think we are all convinced by now that what we eat—or don't eat—is certainly capable of affecting our behavior.

Would it surprise you to know that how a person eats may have something to do with whether or not he becomes a heavy drinker?

Here's an interesting statement from the Bible: "Blessed art thou, O land, when thy king is the son of nobles, and thy princes eat in due season, for strength, and not for drunkenness." Ecclesiastes 10:17.

For strength and not for drunkenness. Is it possible to eat for drunkenness? Well, listen to what happened at Loma Linda University.

Researchers there conducted some experiments with rats. They fed them the typical teenage diet. And it's quite typical for a lot of adults too. Here it is:

Breakfast—doughnuts and coffee. Ten o'clock and three o'clock break—sweet rolls and coffee. Lunch—a hot dog with mustard and pickle relish, a soft drink, apple pie, and coffee. Dinner—spaghetti and meatballs, French garlic bread, green beans, tossed salad, chocolate cake, and coffee. TV snack—a candy bar, cookies, and coffee.

This food, with some common spices added, was all mixed together, dried, and ground into a uniform mix. This would prevent any rats from choosing one food and leaving another.

Then for their drink they were permitted a choice. They could have either water or 10 percent alcohol. They had free access to both.

Another group of rats, for comparison, was fed a diet that was nutritionally adequate and given their choice of the same two drinks.

What happened? The rats fed the teenage diet chose to drink at least five times as much alcohol as did the rats on the adequate diet.

In another study, rats were fed the teenage diet *without* coffee and spices. When coffee was added, their alcohol consumption doubled. When both coffee and spices were added, they drank almost four times as much alcohol as on the diet without coffee and spices.

What do you think of that? Evidently what is on your plate just could have something to do with what you choose to drink. And coffee and spices would seem to be the chief offenders. Along with an inadequate diet that is too low in essential nutrients and too high in sugar.

It was back in 1943 that four researchers in Chile reported on some interesting experiments. Rats were fed a diet deficient in vitamins of the B group—chiefly on white bread. This diet of white bread created a craving for alcohol in the test animals. The researchers concluded that there is a factor in whole-grain bread that "seems to have the specific property of being able to remove the craving for alcohol."

But now we come to something even more vital. What you eat may do more than produce a craving for strong drink. It may also mean that you have less willpower to resist that craving!

Do I mean that what we eat can affect our willpower? Yes, I do.

It takes a very small straw to break the back of willpower. One researcher says that "the irritability resulting from a morning cup of coffee has torpedoed many a resolve to leave off drugs or tobacco."

The same writer points out that within a few moments after eating, drinking, or inhaling, the chemicals we have just taken in are already in the bloodstream exerting an influence over the composition of the proteins and hormones produced in the brain.

Now here is something important. As we have pointed out before, conscience, with which we discriminate between right and wrong, operates through the mind, through the brain. And so conscience is necessarily affected by the quality of the brain tissue.

Is it surprising, then, that moral delinquency can sometimes be linked to eating habits?

I'm not saying the answer is all in good nutrition. Far from it. Yet a researcher in malnutrition does say, "Will is the desire and the power to carry out decisions of reason and conscience. Atrophy of the will has been observed in many ages and places to be the concomitant of prolonged malnutrition."

So the two do often go together!

Ellen White, a writer in whom I have great confidence, said many years ago that tobacco destroys the very sensibilities of the brain with which we discern the wrongness of smoking.

And recent research at the Medical University of South Carolina suggests that even one drink of alcohol can permanently damage the brain. If this research proves to be true, then it means that every time you take a drink of alcohol, brain cells are destroyed—never to be replaced!

Think of it! Brain cells destroyed by alcohol. The finer sensibilities of the brain destroyed by tobacco. And we are beginning to find out more about what other drugs are doing to the brain.

But evidently the harmless-looking food we eat can dull the mind too—and the conscience. And food becomes mighty important when we realize that it can affect the conscience. Because it is with the conscience that we make decisions—decisions that could affect our final destiny.

It's a sobering thought that some of us will lose out in the final day. Not because God has any desire that we should lose out. But because we have put into our bodies things that have dulled the mind and made it difficult and almost impossible to make clear decisions, to discriminate between right and wrong, to make right choices. And yet God has to honor our choices, right or wrong. Otherwise we wouldn't be free.

Don't you long for the day when all of us, if we choose, cured of our rebellion, can be restored to radiant health? I do. Jesus, when He was here, was impatient for that day. That's why He healed so many.

He fed five thousand one day with miracle bread. And I think I know what was in His mind. I think He was looking forward to the day when He could offer them fruit from the tree of life— instead of bread. I'm sure He can hardly wait for that day!

On the very last page of the Bible it says, "Blessed are they that do his commandments, that they may have right to the tree of life, and may enter in through the gates into the city."

Who will have access to the tree? Who will eat its invigorating fruit and never die? Those who have kept God's commandments. Not only His moral law, but His laws of health. Those who have taken care of their bodies. Those who have made right decisions—because their minds have been kept clear enough to make them!

We have a lot to look forward to. And a lot to think about— and some changes to make—in the meantime!

The Vegetarian Thing

What is this vegetarian thing?

Is it a fad for the gullible? The excuse of the weak for despising the strong? The haven of the tenderhearted? A lingering descent into an early grave?

Is it simply the latest Hollywood craze? A scheme to make money?

Or is it the way to health and happiness?

Whether you call it prejudice or preference, convenience or conviction, habit or hang-up—all you have to do is drop your money in the slot, press the button, unwrap your choice—and live by the consequences!

There is an old story about a science professor in a boys' school. He had an uncanny knowledge of animal life. You could show him the bone of an animal, and he would name the animal. You could show him the scale of a fish, and he would not only name the fish but tell you all about its habits. Animal life was his world.

One day the boys decided to play a little trick on the professor. They took the skeleton of a bear and stuffed it. Then they sewed over it the skin of a lion. On its head they fastened the horns of a Texas steer, and on its feet they glued the hooves of a wild buffalo.

They spent a good many nights on the trick, and they did a pretty good job. Then one afternoon when the professor was taking a nap, they tiptoed into his study and set up the monstrosity. From outside the door they let out an unearthly growl such as had never been heard before.

Well, the professor woke up, the story says, tumbled off his cot, and stood bolt upright. His reaction was enough to justify all the time they had spent on the trick. But then through their peepholes they saw a surprising thing. The professor rubbed his eyes, looked at the teeth, the horns, and finally at the split hooves. Then he said, loud enough for the peepholers to hear, "Thank goodness! It's herbivorous, not carnivorous!" And went back to finish his nap.

The professor knew that any animal with horns and split hooves is a vegetarian and would prefer hay or grass to a sleeping professor.

Well, how do *you* react to a *person* who is a vegetarian? If you are like most people you probably consider him harmless, even if you do think he is strangely put together—and go back to your nap.

Vegetarianism, however, is experiencing a surprising new prosperity—largely due to an excellent trend in health education and the health-food movement that is sweeping the country. But people are giving up their steaks for a wide variety of other reasons too—economical, humane, psychological, and spiritual.

One of the most popular reasons—aside from the high cost of meat—is the conviction that the slaughter of animals for food is morally wrong. And then many see the vegetarian way of life as part of an attempt to escape from our mechanized society.

Hollywood, of course, has not escaped the vegetarian bandwagon. Meat seems to be "out" with a great many so-called "in" people. And if we were to do a little table-hopping among the celebrities we would hear some interesting reasons for their choice of diet.

Actress Candice Bergen feels that the slaughter of animals is primitive and cruel. She says, "I was becoming more and more conscious of the insanity around me. Killing animals to feed us seemed to me a part of that insanity. First, it seemed unappetizing and then it became disgusting. Finally, it seemed so primitive, so cruel, really horrid!" She says, "I think I became a vegetarian so I could look animals in the face."

Another actress, Susan St. James, has an interesting angle.

She strongly believes that you can tell a vegetarian by his disposition. She says, "There's a calm that comes over you and a tremendous peace of mind when you're around vegetarians. You relate to animals a lot better, because the animals sense that you're not going to kill them and they give you faith."

Well, do you suppose the animals do sense who their friends are? It does seem inconsistent, doesn't it, to treat animals as family pets and then finally betray them by sending them to the slaughterhouse.

But this matter of the disposition. Is it true that vegetarians are more comfortable to be around? I would hope so, of course—since I happen to be one.

But you decide. Is it possible that to some extent a person absorbs the characteristics of the animals whose flesh he eats? Some think so.

This much we do know. We are, in a sense, what we eat. The cells in our body are constantly being replaced. And those cells have to be made from the food we give our bodies.

We might be shocked if we knew how many top-level decisions, how many committee actions, how many twists in the course of history, have been influenced by what somebody had for dinner.

By the way, as for memorable vegetarians, who is better known than the outstanding critic, George Bernard Shaw? He lived to be 94. And he said, "The enormity of eating scorched, defunct animals becomes impossible the moment it becomes a conscious act, for on such a diet a man cannot do the finest work of which he is capable."

And, still in the past, there was Charles Spurgeon of London, the Billy Graham of the last century. He said, "I have lived on a purely vegetable diet and am a 100 percent better man for it, which convinces me others can do so, too."

And John Wesley, the famed pioneer of the Methodist Church. Did you know that he was a vegetarian? Evidently he was. It is reported that he said, "Thank God, since I gave up the eating of the flesh of animals I have bidden adieu to all the ills my flesh was heir to."

We could go on. Evidently this vegetarian thing is not new.

Well, as I said a few moments ago, I personally am a vegetarian. To be more exact, I am a lacto-ovo-vegetarian. That simply means that my diet is one that includes a limited amount of milk, eggs, and cheese. But I have never knowingly eaten flesh food, fish, or fowl.

Now I suppose that if I were down at the South Pole and there was nothing else to eat, I would eat a piece of meat. And probably if I were shipwrecked and spent a week on a raft, a fish that happened to flop onto that raft would be in as much danger from me as anyone else. But I have never been shipwrecked. And though I have traveled a great deal at home and abroad, by plane and otherwise, and have eaten many, many meals in restaurants of all kinds, I have just never met up with any emergency in which I felt it was necessary to eat flesh food.

Someone is saying, "Pastor Vandeman, you've really missed a lot."

Yes, maybe I have.

One thing I have missed is the risk of contracting a variety of diseases that are evidently have been transmitted to humans through the handling and use of meat.

Ever heard of the science of zoonosis? That's the name of a branch of biological science which has carefully documented 150 diseases that have been transmitted to humans from animals—bacterial, viral, parasitic transmission, or by direct contact.

But you say, "I'm very careful about the quality of the meat I buy."

That may be true, but notice. Nutrition studies have concluded that trichinosis from infected pork is no longer a concern for the general population of this country that it once was—to the credit of the producers in adjusting the food content of the swine and our health departments and cooperation of the meat packing industry. However, recent outbreaks of trichinosis from beef have alarmed these agencies when it was discovered that in 20 percent of the stores that sold beef, some of the beef had been contaminated by the knives and the grinders of the machines that had been cutting up pork. In this way, an outbreak of dreaded trichinosis has at times reared its ugly head again from pork-contaminated beef, for pork, you see, is the source of trichina.

But what about poultry? Isn't it different, you ask? Isn't it safe? An Associated Press dispatch says, "A government panel of scientists has recommended that chickens bearing cancer virus be allowed on the market as long as the birds don't look too repugnant."

And what about fish? Surely they are clean. After all, they take a bath every day.

Well, in Canada's clean rivers it has been discovered that only 1 percent of the fish contain cancer. But 4 percent, four times as much cancer has been found in the fish taken from the Fox River basin that drains the waste and toxic poisons of the Chicago, Illinois, area.

Yes, I think you'll agree, I've missed a lot by being a vegetarian.

Now, a person could become a vegetarian for a variety of reasons. By refusing to eat meat you could protest the violence in our civilization. Or your vegetarianism could be an ecological protest. A vegetarian can be supported by one third the land required to feed a meat eater.

Yes, you could become a vegetarian out of protest. But fortunately there is an even better reason for making the change. It could be your way of responding to God's invitation to eat that which is good. Let me read it:

"Why do you spend money for what is not bread, and your wages for what does not satisfy? Listen diligently to Me, and eat what is good, and let your soul delight itself in abundance." Isaiah 55:2, NKJV.

Well, that's interesting. Foodstuffs that don't give you strength. But most people think that meat gives you strength—that, in fact, you have to have it for strength. Is that true? Listen to this from Dr. Stare of Harvard University: "Lumberjacks may demand plenty of red meat, but that demand rests on habit and not on nutritional or a medical basis."

Habit. But don't you have to have meat for endurance? someone insists.

An article in *Nutrition Today* reports experiments with athletes on various diets. Those on a fat and meat protein diet rode bicycles only 57 minutes. Those on a normal mixed diet rode for one hour, 54 minutes before becoming exhausted. But those on a high carbohydrate diet with no meat rode two hours, 47 minutes. Three times longer than the high fat and meat diet.

I was born in the shadow of Pikes Peak in Colorado. It has always been a mystery to me how anyone could *run* up and down that 14,110-foot peak. But they have a race every year. It's a 28-mile round trip—up and down.

And a friend of mine, Mavis Lindgren, among others, of course, has run that mountain one way two times, and she ran both ways once in 9 hours and 11 minutes. And would you believe it, she is 78 years of age!

Before the age of 62, she had suffered several serious bouts with pneumonia. And in sheer self defense, she changed her health habits and began exercising. Walking and running. Now at 78, she runs 60 miles a week. She's a vegetarian and neither smokes nor drinks. Talk about drive and endurance!

If flesh food is necessary for endurance, then how do we explain the people of Hunza, that interesting Shangri-La north of Pakistan where some men and women live to be well over a hundred years old?

The Hunzakuts for centuries have eaten very little meat of any kind. In recent years, with better access to our western world, they eat more. Their endurance for centuries has been legend. But today, with more of our western food, there have been some disappointing changes in their longevity.

It should be no surprise, then, that the traditional diet of the Hunza people through the centuries almost exactly parallels the original diet that God gave to man in Eden, when man was first created.

Yes, right back at the beginning, God started man out with a new body. And He told him what to put into it. Listen:

"See, I have given you every herb that yields seed which is on the face of all the earth, and every tree whose fruit yields seed; to you it shall be for food." Genesis 1:29, NKJV.

A new body. And how to feed it. What to put into it to keep it operating at peak efficiency. A sort of owner's manual, you see.

And what did God give? He gave fruits, grains, and nuts. And later added vegetables.

Yes, in the beginning, everybody went for natural foods. And those foods kept a person going a long time. Adam lived 950 years. Methuselah lived 969. Many of these people lived three, four, six, or seven hundred years.

Then came the flood of Noah's day. And after the flood, beause the natural foods had all been destroyed, God gave man permission, I believe, as an emergency measure, to eat the flesh of animals. Not all animals, you understand—only certain ones that God designated as fit for food.

But man liked the emergency diet. And he's still eating and liking it. However, it is interesting to note that when man started fooling around with flesh food, things started going downhill immediately, including his life span.

Now we know Jesus ate fish while on earth, and possibly the flesh foods eaten by the humble peasants of Galilee. But with the rising incidence of disease in food animals and the myriad of shots given to counteract disease in these animals, the New Testament counsel to care for our bodies as temples of the Holy Spirit makes good sense.

You see, God has told me that my body is a temple of the Holy Spirit.

"Do you not know that you are the temple of God and that the Spirit of God dwells in you?" 1 Corinthians 3:16, NKJV.

And He has told me not to defile that body.

"If anyone defiles the temple of God, God will destroy him. For the temple of God is holy, which temple you are." 1 Corinthians 3:17, NKJV.

He has told me to eat and drink to the glory of God.

"Therefore, whether you eat or drink, or whatever you do, do all to the glory of God." 1 Corinthians 10:13, NKJV.

I am a Seventh-day Adventist minister, and the longevity of my people, even with only about half of them active vegetarians, yields amazing statistics.

Since 1900, the longevity of the general population in the United States rose 5.6 years. In other words, at age 40 the general population lives 5.6 years longer now than in 1900. But during this same time, the longevity—the life span specifically of the 40-year-old Adventist male—rose to 11 plus years, or 6 years longer than the public in general.

In addition, Seventh-day Adventists experience only one half of the cancer and one half of the heart trouble suffered by the rest of us. That's pretty convincing evidence that their lifestyle as documented by the New Testament is worth considering, wouldn't you say?

What about the nation's number one killer—heart disease? The World Health Organization Expert Committee on Coronary Heart Disease Prevention has said as recently as 1983 that in their opinion the relationship between diet, blood cholesterol, and heart attacks is a *causal* relationship. Did you notice that word *causal?*

Seldom has a scientific organization of such prestige said that diet and blood cholesterol can be the cause of heart trouble. Evidently there is a growing awareness in the best of scientific circles that a meat-and-egg-laden fatty diet is not only suspect but is to a large extent the culprit in robbing us of vital heart support.

Well, some of you may decide to go out to the kitchen after reading this and clean out your refrigerator. And for that reaction you are to be commended. But, I say, be careful. Be sure that you make the transition in your diet slowly and intelligently. Be sure that as you leave off flesh proteins you replace them with other adequate vegetable proteins. This is important.

I wish I could invite you all home to dinner—one at a time, you understand, not all at once. I'd like you to enjoy with me a big baked russet potato, perhaps with sour cream and chives. Then one of those delicious protein entrees made from grains or soybeans or nuts. Not heavy—just light and delicious. My wife Nellie is absolutely unsurpassed at making them. Then a lightly cooked vegetable or two. An attractive green salad. Some good whole-wheat bread. And a simple, light dessert. I tell you, this is the life.

You see, the vegetarian diet is certainly wholesome and nutritious, but it can be delectable as well. And you feel so much better living this way.

And now let me close this chapter with an unusual statement by the distinguished Intersociety Commission for Heart Disease Resources. They said, "Salvation"—that is, success in lowering the risk of heart disease—"Salvation is largely dependent upon your personal decision." You see, success in lowering the risk of heart disease, according to these experts, is largely dependent upon your personal decision.

A personal decision—a commitment. And I would like to add to that statement a commitment of dedication. And that is what it can be for you now. If you have already made a commitment to the Lord Jesus Christ as your Saviour, wouldn't you like today to make a new kind of commitment? You have given Him your heart. Wouldn't you like to give Him your body, too? Wouldn't you like to tell your Lord that, beginning now, you want your commitment to Him to be complete, mind and body, without any reservation?

The New Medicine

Norman Cousins, then editor of *The Saturday Review*, was in a New York Hospital. He was suffering from a mysterious joint and connective tissue disease that specialists agreed was incurable. They said he would almost certainly be permanently crippled.

So Norman Cousins did some research of his own. He knew that negative emotions are harmful. Now, as he read, he was convinced that positive emotions—such as common, everyday joy of living—could heal. He was convinced, too, that the prescription drugs he was taking were probably harming more than helping. So he decided that all he needed was some high doses of intravenous vitamin C and something to laugh about.

First he asked for a projector in his room, so that he could watch some old "Candid Camera" television films every few hours. Then, very soon, he left the hospital, took his "Candid Camera" reruns and his vitamin C to a hotel room, and set about, with the approval of his physician, to heal himself.

Today Norman Cousins plays Bach fugues, tennis, and the typewriter as well as ever!

Now he's not suggesting, nor am I, that his treatment would work for everyone, or that he wouldn't have got well anyway. But his experience does demonstrate the beneficial effects of just plain laughing. It also demonstrates that sometimes a patient, under a physician's guidance, has to heal *himself*.

This is interesting. Because that was 1964. Today, in the eighties, something is happening called the "new medicine."

And the new medicine is turning over to the patient more and more of the responsibility for the healing process. And this is good.

It's about time something like this happened, of course. It's true that we've seen one medical miracle after another. And we wouldn't for a moment want to be without them. Yet these miracles of modern medicine have contributed to the current medical crisis. Antibiotics have been overused, and now, as a result, we have dangerous drug-resisting bacteria. So we have stronger and stronger drugs—some with deadly side effects. Ingenious surgery and life-support systems make it possible to keep people alive longer—*and we're so thankful*. But all this is at astronomical cost.

Not only that, medical practice is more and more specialized. House calls, with most doctors, are long since out. Malpractice jitters lead the fearful to order more and more tests the patient may not need. And, in too many instances, the distance between a physician's hello and goodbye is getting shorter and shorter. Some patients hardly know whether they are being treated by a physician or a questionnaire. A computer now can play the role of psychiatrist, I am told.

There are happy exceptions to all this, you understand. There are thousands of dedicated physicians who are just as interested in their patients as the old-time family doctor ever was. They are committed to the highest standards of medical care. They give of their strength way beyond the call of duty. There are thousands of these, I say. Many of them are my friends. Many of them, with their financial support, help to make the "It Is Written" telecast possible. They do this because they know that true healing must touch the spiritual needs of men and women as well as the physical. So nothing I have said, or will say, in these pages is intended as a wholesale indictment of the medical profession. Far from it. We are talking about trends. And, of course, wherever the trends are disturbing, the exceptions stand out the brighter!

But back to these trends. There is another problem. According to George Leonard, writing in *New West* magazine, "Doctor-prescribed drugs . . . have become one of the nation's major causes of death. Adverse drug reactions probably total at least 3 million a year. Estimates of hospital deaths due to drugs range up to 140,000 a year." But he says that even if you take "the rather conservative figure of 29,000 deaths from the Boston Collaborative Drug Study, you will have adverse drug reaction as the eleventh most deadly killer in the United States, just behind bronchitis, emphysema, and asthma."

But then, he says, we must "combine these drug reactions *in* hospitals with the estimated 300,000 people *admitted* to hospitals every year because of doctor-prescribed drugs." And then there are the side effects of surgery and radiation, and, of course, the inevitable human error on the part of everburdened hospital employees—even though they do their best.

Evidently hospitals *can be* dangerous places.

The alternative to all this, the alternative we have to activate with all possible speed—is to turn our attention to preventing disease instead of just trying to cure it.

And that presents a problem, because most physicians today have been trained only to cure disease. Many of them know comparatively little about prevention. The kind of therapy they have been trained to give, and we have been trained to accept, is the doctor-knows-best variety—in which the physician prescribes and the patient helplessly places himself in the hands of the professional healer. Again, there are exceptions. I know physicians who have been practicing preventive medicine a long time.

Now, of course, if you happen to have appendicitis, or if you get hit by a truck, you can be mighty thankful for the nearest hospital, and for what some are now calling the old medicine. That's the sort of thing the old medicine handles best.

Once more, don't misunderstand me. I am not in any way downgrading the triumphs and the accomplishments of modern conventional medicine. Gone, for instance, are the great infectious diseases—smallpox, cholera, typhoid, diphtheria, yellow fever, tuberculosis, and polio. At least they have been cut down to where they can be easily managed.

But what do we have in their place? We have a whole list of what we might call "civilized" diseases—diseases largely caused by our modern lifestyle. And they are hard to treat. You know what they are—cardiovascular diseases, cancer, lung diseases, diabetes, nervous disorders—and on and on.

Do you realize that in spite of all the strides of modern medicine, "some 80 percent of a doctor's work consists of treating minor complaints and giving reassurance. Common colds, minor injuries, gastrointestinal upsets, back pain, arthritis, and psychoneurotic anxiety states account for the vast majority of visits to clinics and doctors' offices."

Says Dr. Philip R. Lee, Professor of Social Medicine at the University of California School of Medicine, "If all abuse of tobacco, alcohol, and automobiles could be magically erased with the snap of a finger, at least half of all hospital beds in this country would suddenly be empty."

But he's talking about problems of lifestyle. He's not talking about unavoidable scourges. He's talking about things we could do something about—if we would!

But the physician can't. The physician can recommend. He can urge. He can warn. But he can't follow his patient around day and night and knock the cigarette out of his hand every time he lights one up. He can't make him get enough sleep. He can't force him to get up out of his easy chair and take a walk. He can't eat dinner with him every night and push him back from the table when he's had enough to eat. He can't go through the refrigerator every day—or go along to the supermarket and monitor what goes into the shopping cart!

Do you see? If so many diseases are caused by our lifestyle, then whose responsibility is the prevention of disease? The physician can counsel. But doesn't the patient have to be his own doctor most of the time? If the bathroom scale tells him he's gaining weight, does he have to wait for his doctor, at his next scheduled appointment, to tell him he should eat less?

Is it surprising, then, that the new medicine, realizing all this, is saying that the responsibility for maintaining health must be shifted largely to the individual? It's the patient, not the doctor, who is in charge most of the time. Most of the time he is treating himself—by his lifestyle, by his habits, by the exercise he gets or doesn't get, by the number of hours he allows for sleep, by the stress under which he permits himself to live.

Individual effort, then, the new medicine is saying, is the answer to the high cost of curing disease—because it is the best way to prevent it.

According to this new concept, your life and health seldom depend upon drugs or surgical techniques. Most of the time your health and how long you live depend on factors that you yourself can control.

"Stop smoking," says the new medicine, "and you stand to gain two to twelve years. Moderate your intensely competitive personality and you gain up to eight years." You can *choose* to be healthy, you can choose to live longer—because you can choose your lifestyle. Dying in the crash of a commercial plane may be out of your control. But you can choose not to die of a heart attack because of faulty living habits. That is in your power!

The new medicine is called holistic medicine, because it deals with the whole man—not just his body, but his mind and his emotions and his lifestyle as well. And, of course, as we've already seen, that's the kind of healing Jesus practiced. Not only did He heal people's physical maladies. He healed their guilt. He told them their illness was the result of their sin. He told them to sin no more. He said to one man who was brought to Him for healing, "Take heart, son; your sins are forgiven." Matthew 9:2, NIV.

And to another He said, "Stop sinning or something worse may happen to you." John 5:14, NIV.

The healing that Jesus practiced was never separated from His compassion and from His teaching. He loved men and women. He sympathized with them. He listened to them. But He did not heal promiscuously, leaving men by their wrong habits to make themselves ill again. He taught them how to live. He reached down to heal—but also to lift.

Dr. Art Ulene, on NBC television, told how the White Memorial Hospital clinicians in Los Angeles are practicing holistic medicine. He used their treatment of arthritis as an example. True, they use aspirin, and they use cortisone injections. But they also use physical therapy. And they deal with the emotions of their patients.

Arthritis, said Dr. Ulene, is much like surgery. The surgeon may perform a perfect operation. But if the patient has no will to live, he dies. So at the White Memorial they listen to their patients. They let them talk about their feelings. A person who has arthritis is often depressed, afraid he will not be able to carry on, afraid he will become a burden to his family. One patient, with tears streaming down her cheeks, said, "Nobody has ever listened to me before!"

Dr. Ulene gave this bit of counsel to anyone who has arthritis: "Don't think of yourself as an arthritic. You're a *person* who happens to have arthritis."

A person first. A patient second. That's holistic medicine!

So far in this discussion we haven't found anything to criticize in the new medicine. Certainly in treating the whole man, in shifting more of the responsibility for healing to the patient and in placing the major emphasis on prevention of disease, it has to be on the right track.

I wish that were all the story. But unfortunately it isn't. The truth is that I don't know when I've seen such a blend of the good and the dangerous—with the two so intertwined that it is difficult to sort them out. So much that is commendable. And so much that shouts, Beware!

So let's take a look. And I think you'll see why it troubles me.

The new medicine, according to one magazine, "is the creation of a large and colorful cast of characters, ranging from established medical professionals to psychic healers and Indian shamans." The magazine admits that the new concept "will draw its share of charlatans," and that "trivial, faddist practices will masquerade under the name 'holistic.' " It publishes some guidelines on "how to tell the healers from the wheeler-dealers." One of its cautions is that "the familiar 'doctor knows best' attitude should not become 'your hypnotist knows best.' "

Hypnosis, for instance, under any label, involves the surrender of a person's will to that of another. And that is always dangerous. To surrender the will is to abdicate the power of choice. It is to let another person, another entity, make your decisions.

The conscience operates through the mind. Anything that dulls the mind dulls the conscience. Anything that inactivates the mind inactivates the conscience. Yet it is with the conscience that we make moral decisions, decisions that affect our eternal destiny. Can it ever be safe to turn the conscience over to another—and perhaps with it our destiny?

So I think you can see why I was concerned when I read a partial list of techniques that are being used in the new medicine. Listen:

"Self-healing with visualization, herbal studies, physical fitness and consciousness training, applied meditation, iridology (reading the eyes for knowledge of internal body conditions), auto-hypnosis, reflexology, massage and centering, and the psychic process of healing."

It isn't too difficult, is it, to find the telltale footprints of hypnosis and psychic healing in that list of techniques? So I'm troubled. I feel I must say, "Be careful. Be on guard." Because Solomon, the wise man, says, "Guard your heart more than any treasure." Proverbs 4:23, NEB.

Guard your heart—your mind. Don't let anybody have it. Don't let anybody tamper with it. That's good counsel. And never have we needed it more than today!

The mind once surrendered to another is more easily breached the second time. There may be apparent healing. But the mind has been weakened. It is never so strong again. Can we afford healing—at that price?

I say again, You have an enemy. He's an angel fallen. He's out to destroy you any way he can. Your mind is his target. He wants your mind. He wants your will. He wants control!

Hypnosis is one of his favorite tools. And he tries to slip it in under a thousand harmless-sounding labels. With his subtle philosophies, so often unrecognized, he infiltrates the beautiful concept of holistic healing and robs it of its power.

In true holistic healing, the kind that Jesus practiced, there is no control of the mind. There is no attempt to seize a man's will, or to suspend the operation of his conscience. There is no tampering with man's power of choice. The mind and the will and the conscience are free at all times. Jesus often *freed* men from outside control. But never did He *use* it!

But Jesus knew what we are so slow to learn—that there is

no true and lasting healing of the whole man unless it gives priority to his relationship to God. A man alienated from his God—is he a happy man? Is he a healthy man? A man full of guilt that he can't erase, and that no man can heal—is he a man in optimum health? A man distressed and depressed and oppressed with burdens too heavy to carry, burdens only his Lord can lift—does he have peace of mind? Has he experienced true healing, healing of the whole man? No, friend. No.

That's why Jesus placed forgiveness first and healing of the body second. He had His priorities straight. He knew how heavy the load of guilt can be. He knew that there were thousands, then and now, who wouldn't even care about healing of the body if only their guilt could be healed. That's why He said, "Come to me, all you who are weary and burdened, and I will give you rest. Take my yoke upon you and learn from me, for I am gentle and humble in heart, and you will find rest for your souls. For my yoke is easy and my burden is light." Matthew 11:28-30, NIV.

"Come to me . . . and I will give you rest." No finer prescription has ever been written!

Quitting Can Be Tough

For two hours a hostage was held, sometimes at gunpoint, atop the tallest building in Los Angeles. Television viewers were fed live coverage of the developing drama from a circling helicopter.

The man with the gun, of course, had a demand. He had left a message in his briefcase on the fifty-fifth floor. Either his message must be read over local radio, or he would jump.

What was his message? That's the story.

Dolphin Lair was only twenty-one. He was a school custodian, as his father had been before him. Ever since he was a small boy he had wanted to do the same work his father did— meeting people, helping people, learning from people.

But two months earlier his father had died of throat cancer. "In eight months this year," Dolphin said, "I saw my father go from a big strong man to a small, shriveled up . . . snail. You can imagine how he looked; like a skeleton with skin color painted on.

"The last day before he died I held him in my arms and carried him to bed. He mumbled something to mother. He wanted to pray, but he didn't know how because he wasn't religious. My mother told him just to say what was in his head. He passed away during the night."

Smoking had done it. Two packs a day.

During the months that his father lay dying, Dolphin began visiting the public library to learn all he could about cancer and tobacco. He memorized Webster's definition of nicotine: "A poi-

sonous alkaloid, the chief active principle of tobacco."
"Poisonous," he kept repeating to himself, as he watched his
father die.

He talked to anyone who would listen. But that wasn't
enough. He called the federal Food and Drug Administration to
ask why cigarettes were not declared a poisonous drug. He
wrote to his congresswoman. He kept asking doctors why they
didn't do anything about it.

It seemed nobody would do anything. He said, "People sit
around every day, saying 'I'm gonna do this, I'm gonna do that,'
and they never do it. But they could have done it." He said,
"You can't depend on anyone else. Parents die. Eventually you
have to do it yourself."

He called the *Times*. He called the *Herald Examiner*. He
called several radio and TV stations. They all told him that one
unknown person expressing his opinion wasn't news.

It was then that his father died.

Now he was desperate. He had to get his message across.
Other people must not die as his father had died—without
knowing. If his message wasn't newsworthy, he would have to
make it newsworthy. He called a television newsroom and
threatened to jump off a roof unless someone came out to talk to
him. The woman on the other end of the line, he said, told him
she didn't have time to bother with him. She said, "Go ahead
and jump," and then hung up. No one in the newsroom would
own up to saying that, but that's the way he remembered it.

That set him thinking. If Jesus had sacrificed His life to help
people, why couldn't he do the same? He had to get people to
listen!

He couldn't just jump off his own roof. That wouldn't draw
enough attention. He found out the United California Bank
building was the tallest in town. He thought about it for nearly
a week, with no sleep. Was he going insane? Or was this something he had to do?

He loved his wife and their small daughter. That made it
hard. But on the morning of December 6 he dressed in a light
blue vested suit and white tie, and went downtown with his
wife to buy Christmas presents for their daughter. He had

slipped into his pocket a plastic starter's pistol, the kind they use at track meets. It would keep anyone from grabbing him and holding him back.

His wife knew nothing of his plans. He gave her the go-cart and dolls they had purchased for their daughter, kissed her goodbye, and started walking toward the UCB building. He says, "I felt scary."

He had no intention of taking a hostage. But the top two floors were locked. The man with the keys wouldn't grant him admission, so he pulled out the plastic pistol and demanded to be taken to the roof.

His hostage soon realized the young man had no desire to harm him. He listened, not without sympathy, to the young man's story, and urged him not to jump. Dolphin says he owes his life to his hostage.

Finally, over the little transistor radio he had brought with him, he heard his three-page message being broadcast. That was all he wanted. He surrendered quietly to police. He was charged with kidnapping.

And then suddenly, in almost no time, the media descended upon him. There they were—the reporters. Cameras were rolling. A team of *Times* reporters were scrambling to piece the story together. He says, "All those news guys I had tried to talk to before were down there. All sorts of high class people were interested. They all wanted to talk to me. I asked them why they didn't talk to me in the beginning."

Dolphin realizes he didn't go about it the right way. But he says his mother has stopped smoking now. She wouldn't before. And he's had quite a few letters from people saying they've stopped smoking because of what he did. And he says, "If that's true, then it was worth it, even if I go to jail!"

Most smokers want to quit. Most smokers have tried to quit. Most smokers have failed.

For that reason no-smoking clinics are springing up all over the country. And no doubt all of them have helpful features. But the one I am most familiar with, and one I can highly recommend, is one conducted by the Seventh-day Adventists. It is known as the Breathe Free Plan to Stop Smoking. Watch for it when it comes to your area. You can't go wrong in attending.

One reason the Adventist program has been so sucessful is that a need for divine aid in kicking the habit is emphasized.

That's why Alcoholics Anonymous has succeeded. Every AA member recognizes his need of divine power to overcome his drinking problem.

And believe me, there is no substitute for divine power. Anyone who tries to break a habit without it is attempting something almost impossible. I say "almost," because some individuals with very strong willpower have been able to do it on their own. But I don't need to tell you that most people who have a smoking problem, a drinking problem, a drug problem, or even an overweight problem, have very little willpower!

You see, it's very difficult to scare a person into quitting. Smokers know the facts. You hear them and read them and see them all the time, as I do. It isn't difficult to scare a person into *wanting* to quit. But quitting is something else.

Back to the story of Dolphin for just a moment. You recall he was happy that his mother, because of what he had done, had stopped smoking. That is, he thought she had. But his mother, later, told a reporter over the phone, "Well, not really, I've cut back, but I still smoke. I used to smoke a pack every day and a half; now it's a pack every two days." And then she added, "But I sure don't smoke in front of Dolphin. I have too much respect for him to do that."

Sound familiar? Do you know some smokers who could identify with that kind of behavior? Cutting back? Yes. Being careful? Yes. But quitting?

Quitting can be difficult. Only the one who has tried and failed repeatedly knows how difficult. Tomorrow seems not to exist, but only the pleasure of the moment, the craving, the cigarette in your hand. And while once more you push quitting into tomorrow, promising not to ignore it then, the tomorrows keep slipping away. Cause and effect keep on playing tag. No angel stops by to blow out the match. And the cry for help, though silent, crowds closer and closer to despair. You wonder if there is any hope for a smoker like you. And you wonder if anyone cares.

And yes, it may be I'm talking about you!

Smokers are not dumb. They are intelligent people. They know what their habit is doing to them. But it seems they can't quit. There are those who will even smoke through a hole in their throat—when part of their throat has had to be cut away by the surgeon's knife. Imagine!

The ones who quit and really stay quit are usually those who quit for moral reasons.

But you say, "Are there moral reasons?"

Let me ask you that question. Isn't it wrong to kill yourself little by little? Isn't it wrong to set an example in something that damages the body? Isn't it wrong to smoke in the presence of those who don't want to smoke—forcing them to breathe the same poisoned air? And isn't it wrong to destroy the body that God asks us to take care of?

I say again, God will permit us to destroy ourselves, if that is what we choose to do. He does not force us to take care of our bodies. But I think you can see that taking care of our bodies *is* a moral issue.

Quitting can be tough. Anyone who is trying to kick a habit can identify with the apostle Paul. Evidently he experienced feelings of frustration much like yours. He said, "My own behaviour baffles me. For I find myself doing what I really loathe but not doing what I really want to do. . . . I often find that I have the will to do good, but not the power. That is, I don't accomplish the good I set out to do, and the evil I don't really want to do I find I am always doing. . . . It is an agonising situation, and who can set me free from the prison of this mortal body?" Romans 7:15-24, Phillips.

Ever feel like that? But Paul found a way out. He says, "I thank God there is a way out through Jesus Christ our Lord." Verse 25.

Yes, Jesus is the way out. When you keep on doing what you don't want to do—and you can't quit—He's the only way out!

So instead of trying to frighten you with all the terrible things that happen to smokers—and alcoholics—and drug addicts—I just want to lift up the Saviour. He's the way out!

Habits are so tricky. They slip in while you're not looking.

They sneak in by the back door. They make their way in like Trojan horses. And then you can't get them out.

We have an understanding Lord, a sympathetic Saviour. He knows that addiction is not always deliberate. Sometimes a physician prescribes a drug for a legitimate temporary need. And then, without ever being intended, addiction follows.

God understands. He is sympathetic. But that doesn't mean He wants us to be slaves to a habit—any habit. Jesus said He came "to preach deliverance to the captives." Luke 4:18.

And He said, "So if the Son sets you free, you will be free indeed." John 8:36, NIV.

And the apostle Paul said, "For sin shall not be your master." Romans 6:14, NIV.

Those are the promises. And you can count on them. They're meant for you personally!

It's easy to give way to a feeling of hopelessness when you've tried and failed so many times. The knowledge of broken promises, broken resolutions, is frustrating. It's depressing. It's easy to feel that no one cares. But look to Jesus. He cares. And He has not failed. His strength has not been diminished one whit by your failure!

So don't despair. All the pledges in the world may not be strong enough to break the chains of habit. But Jesus can. And He will—if you ask Him.

You may not be able to control your feelings, your cravings, your desires. But you can *choose* to quit. You still have your will. And you need to understand the true force of the will. It may be weakened by misuse, or by disuse. But you can choose to be free. Even though you have no power to carry out your choice, you can still make that choice. And when you do, He will supply the power. And you will be free!

So don't look at circumstances. Don't look at your own weakness. Don't look at the power of temptation. Look to Jesus. Tell Him your need. Know that He is able. Know that He cares. He cares as if you were the only one in the world who needed His healing, lifting, saving power at this moment!

From the hearts of millions rises the silent cry for help, for freedom from the persistent, stubborn slavery of a habit that will not let them go, for Someone to break the chains they cannot break. And the Saviour hears each one. Not one is missed.

And He has more than sympathy for the man or woman who is struggling with a habit. He doesn't say, "God bless you. Keep trying." He is able to do something about it. He is able to break the chains. That's why He came to this world to live as a man. Said the angel who announced His mission, "Thou shalt call his name Jesus: for he shall save his people from their sins." Matthew 1:21.

And the apostle Jude said it this way: "To him who is able to keep you from falling and to present you before his glorious presence without fault and with great joy." Jude 24, NIV.

Is it only because Jesus is the Son of God, because He has divine power, that He is able to break the chains? No. It is more than that. The apostle Paul says, "For we do not have a high priest who is unable to sympathize with our weaknesses, but we have one who has been tempted in every way, just as we are—yet was without sin." Hebrews 4:15, NIV.

Jesus walked the same planet that we walk. He met every temptation that we meet. He knows the power and cunning of the tempter as we have never known it. He struggled with that enemy every day of His life—and came off a Conqueror. Scarred? Yes. But not contaminated. Continually harrassed—but never once defeated!

He met the enemy in the wilderness above Jordan—and gained the victory over appetite. And certainly that includes victory over addiction to tobacco and alcohol and drugs and whatever. He did it so that that victory might be yours!

He carried that victory through to the Garden of Gethsemane. And He might have turned back. He might have given up. That was the almost overwhelming temptation. But He didn't. Because of you!

He carried that victory through to the cross. And still He could have turned back. He could have come down from the cross—and let you remain a slave to habit, a slave to sin. But Love couldn't do it! Love couldn't turn back!

With a Love like that, with a Saviour like that, why wait another moment to let Him make His victory yours?

Healing for a Price

When all the reports are in and your physician has reluctantly told you the truth, when suddenly you aren't sure that
you will ever see another summer, when you are jolted into
near shock by the realization that time for you is shorter than
you have ever dreamed, when it seems you can almost see the
figure of death turning in at your driveway, and you feel its
cold breath in your face—what then?

Dr. David Duffie, a friend of mine, was serving at a mission
station in South America when it happened. It was in the early
days of his work as a physician.

He had thought his high fever was just a bad case of the flu.
But on its second day he painfully turned over in bed and asked
his wife Daisy to get a certain big medical book and look up
under "bubonic plague." She did, and read aloud. Everything
checked!

She read on silently. "Little hope after patient is in coma
stage," the book said. "Coma deepens until death." She knew
all too well that bubonic plague was usually fatal. But there
was some hope. The book said, "Sulfadiazine in large doses
sometimes helpful. . . . Antibubonic serum, if given early in the
course of the disease."

Antibubonic serum! Of course! She fairly leaped to her feet.
She would start the sulfa at once. She would cable Lima for the
serum. Dr. Potts would come from Lima. Everything would be
all right!

The cablegram read, "Dr. Duffie. Bubonic plague. Send
antibubonic serum. Urgent. Please reply."

Then they waited. But nothing happened. The fever didn't drop. The serum didn't arrive. There was no word whatever from Dr. Potts. Two days later she sent a second cable.

Later they would learn that the first cable was never received. The second was delivered and signed for by a maid—who put it in a dresser drawer where it wasn't discovered for two days.

On Tuesday afternoon there seemed to be a change. David was quieter, in less pain, and could sleep a little. Daisy was encouraged—until she realized what was really happening. He was slipping into a coma. And she remembered what the book had said—little hope after that.

At 2:00 p.m. the clinic personnel met for special prayer for their doctor. Then Noel, the Argentine nurse, took his little Ford and started for their secondary school seven kilometers away. He would bring back a group of ministers and teachers for a prayer and anointing service, as specified in the Bible by the apostle James. You may recall the words: "Is any sick among you? Let him call for the elders of the church; and let them pray over him, anointing him with oil in the name of the Lord: And the prayer of faith shall save the sick, and the Lord shall raise him up; and if he have committed sins, they shall be forgiven him." James 5:14, 15.

In the meantime Daisy was keeping her lonely vigil at her husband's bedside, wondering why help had not come. There was a knock at the door. It was Marcilino with word of an emergency at the clinic. And Noel, the nurse, was gone—on his way to the school.

She left the boy to sit by the bed with his hand on the doctor's pulse, telling him to report instantly if there was any change.

The emergency proved to be very serious, and it was forty-five minutes later when she rushed back into the house. She found Marcilino sitting on the sofa in the living room nonchalantly leafing through a *National Geographic* magazine. For a moment she was very upset at this seeming disregard of her instructions. The next moment she was terrified at what it might mean. Why was Marcilino in the living room? Had her husband died while she was gone? Why hadn't the boy called her?

Marcilino seemed utterly mystified by her outbreak of emotion. Hesitatingly he tried to answer her questions. "The doctor told me to go out," he said simply.

"The doctor told you? The doctor hasn't spoken for two days!"

She couldn't say another word. Tremblingly she pushed open the closed bedroom door, afraid of what she would find.

The bed was empty. In front of the dresser stood David, fully dressed, his stethoscope in hand!

She gasped, "David Duffie, what are you doing?"

And he answered pleasantly, "Oh, thought I'd better go over to the clinic and make rounds. Haven't seen the patients for several days, have I? What day is it, anyway?"

So it was that when Noel returned from the school with the group of troubled teachers, they met in the consultation room at the clinic, with Dr. Duffie at the desk—not for an anointing service, but for a time of special thanksgiving!

And listen to this. Noel had arrived at the school with the sad news of the doctor's condition at 2:20, and immediately the teachers had dropped to their knees in prayer.

And Marcilino, at the doctor's bedside, had kept careful notes. This is what he had written: "2:20, doctor turned over in bed. 2:25, he asked me what I wanted and told me I could go."

What do you think of that? Does our Lord still heal? Of course He does!

And millions would agree with me. Belief in divine healing—or perhaps I should say in supernatural healing—has today achieved a considerable popularity. Healers are springing up everywhere, it seems.

There are those who seem to feel that divine healing is available at any time on demand—whether or not any real emergency exists. There are even those who see it as a way to beat the high cost of medical and hospital care. Don't bother going to the doctor. Just pray!

And unfortunately there are those who seem to think of healing as a sort of show to be run and rerun—just to demonstrate what God can do.

But God is not in show business. Nor is He in competition with the doctors. Seldom does God step in to do miraculously what we are able to do for ourselves. He acts when there is a need.

It's in situations like that of Dr. Duffie—when there is nothing any man can do, when there is nowhere else to turn, when the need is desperate—it's then that God delights to step in!

Some of you may be facing such a situation at this moment. You've been to doctors. You've been to specialists. Wisely or unwisely you've tried everything suggested by your friends. You've found no help. The outlook is not good.

Desperate to regain a hold on life, you've turned to prayer. You've prayed. Others have prayed. You've gone to this group and that group for help. But nothing has happened. God is supposed to heal, isn't He? Hasn't He said He would? Then why doesn't He?

I want to say something now that may shock you. But stay with me and you'll see why I say it. Listen. *There are places you could go and be healed—temporarily healed, apparently healed. You might experience an undeniable miracle. But the price is too high!*

True, you might not have a hospital bill to pay—or a surgeon or an anesthetist. You might have no scars upon your body. But the cost might be astronomical. You might have sold yourself into slavery. And the scars upon your mind and your conscience might cost you your eternal life!

Let me illustrate. A patient appeared at the door of a healer who had been making some rather striking claims in newspaper ads. She told the healer that the doctors had diagnosed her as having a serious blood disease, possibly leukemia.

The healer replied, "I'm not a medical doctor. I treat with the mind and use hypnosis. The medical profession doesn't have a cure for leukemia. But we have cured leukemia. We have cured cancer, even terminal cancer.

"Lend me your mind," said the healer, "to remove the debris and get your mind functioning properly."

Did you notice? "Lend me your mind." The mind must first be surrendered as part of the price of healing!

The price is too high. You may feel better. Symptoms may have disappeared temporarily. You may be able to walk without crutches. But your mind has been made more susceptible to outside control. The locks on the door of your mind have been jimmied. And now anything can happen!

Of course not all false healers will tell you so openly that the surrender of your mind is a part of the price you pay!

Am I suggesting that not all supernatural healing comes from God? Yes, I am. Am I suggesting that such a beautiful thing as healing—something that seems so right—could sometimes be wrong? Yes, I am. Let me put it bluntly. There are times when healing could be lethal!

You see, as long as people are ill, as long as people seek healing, there will always be ambitious men and women who will step in and try to take advantage of the market. They know that anyone who holds out any hope of cure for the incurable can get a following.

But I wonder if you realize that much of today's healing is strangely unlike that of Jesus. For instance, not once did Jesus advertise His healing powers. Sometimes He even told those He healed not to make it known.

Not once did Jesus say, "There'll be a healing service tonight at 7:30. Come and be healed." He healed when and where there was a need. He didn't make show business out of His healing!

Not once did Jesus try to build up a personality cult around Himself, or take His followers' money to build up a personal empire. When the people wanted to make Him king, He quietly slipped away.

Not once did Jesus *command* His Father to heal. He commanded the demons to leave their victims. But He didn't command His Father to do anything. Should we?

And not once was there noise and confusion and disorder in His meetings. The demons, when He commanded them to come out, sometimes noisily protested and threw their victims to the ground. But that was the work of demons—not the work of Jesus!

We ought not to be surprised at the widespread abuse and perversion of the gift of healing in our day. Jesus indicated that many a miracle with which He would have nothing to do would be worked in His name. Speaking of the day of judgment, He said, "Not everyone who says to me, 'Lord, Lord,' will enter the kingdom of heaven but only he who does the will of my Father who is in heaven. Many will say to me on that day, 'Lord, Lord, did we not prophesy in your name, and in your name drive out demons and perform many miracles?' Then I will tell them plainly, 'I never knew you. Away from me, you evildoers!'" Matthew 7:21-23, NIV.

Think of it! Prophecies made in the name of Jesus. Demons cast out in His name. Miracles worked in His name. But the Lord Jesus refuses to be identified with them!

Unquestionably there are counterfeit miracles. Jesus said that "false Christs and false prophets will appear and perform great signs and miracles." Matthew 24:24, NIV.

And in the book of Revelation we read of "spirits of demons performing miraculous signs." Revelation 16:14, NIV.

But am I sure that the false miracles of our day will include healing? I can't conceive of its being otherwise. I can't conceive of Satan, the enemy of God, missing the chance to deceive on that point.

Tell me. Didn't Jesus spend more time healing than teaching? Didn't most of His miracles involve healing? Then if Satan wants to counterfeit the work of Christ—and of course he does—then wouldn't healing be at the top of his list?

Jesus said concerning His true followers, "They will place their hands on sick people, and they will get well." Mark 16:18, NIV.

Then won't Satan try to do it too?

Evidently the risk of being deceived is very great. We need to step carefully. We need to be cautious. But how can we tell whether a miracle of healing is genuine or counterfeit?

There will be times when we can't—if we look only at the miracle itself. But here's a good rule: If you want to evaluate the healing, listen to the sermon; listen to what is being said, what is being taught. If you hear the Scriptures misused, distorted, contradicted, then no matter how spectacular the miracle, it isn't from God. Said the prophet Isaiah, "To the law and to the testimony: if they speak not according to this word, it is because there is no light in them." Isaiah 8:20.

That's the way to tell. Measure what you hear—and what you see—by the Word of God!

The tragedy is that too many *look* only at the miracle—and then *believe* everything they hear. They reason that the teaching must be true because they saw a miracle. And that's the way millions are trapped in false teaching. That's the way millions are encouraged to disobey God. That's the way millions will be lost!

My heart aches for the man who takes a promise of God out of its context, asks for healing, and then, if he isn't healed, feels that God has broken His word.

For instance, Jesus said, "Ask whatever you wish, and it will be given you." John 15:7, NIV.

Just ask whatever you wish, and God will give it to you. That's what it says, isn't it? And one dear man, when he wasn't healed, couldn't understand. He was dumbfounded when he was told that there were conditions to answered prayer. He couldn't see anything conditional about those words. And he said hopelessly, "Then that cancels out everything in the Bible. If those words aren't true, then nothing God says is true!"

But let's read the entire verse, instead of just part of it as we did before. Listen again: "If you remain in me and my words remain in you, ask whatever you wish, and it will be given you." John 15:7, NIV.

That's different, isn't it? It has an *if.* "If you remain in me."

What does it mean to remain in Christ? Verse 10 tells us: "If you obey my commands, you will remain in my love, just as I have obeyed my Father's commands and remain in his love."

Don't you see? If God were to give us anything we choose to ask *while we are disobeying Him*, it would only encourage us in disobedience, wouldn't it? We'd think we are all right. Because after all, didn't God heal us?

Jesus prayed in Gethsemane, "My Father, if it is possible, may this cup be taken from me." Matthew 26:39, NIV.

But He added these words: "Yet not as I will, but as you will."

If those words were appropriate on the lips of Jesus, how much more appropriate they are on ours!

If we ask for healing and we are not healed, does it mean that

God doesn't care? Does it mean He doesn't love us? Does it mean He wants us to die?

No! A thousand times No!

But can we expect to be healed while we go around mad at God for not healing us? Can we expect to be healed while we make healing a condition of our loving and serving Him? We can't bargain with God. We aren't members of a union negotiating a contract—no healing, no work!

If we have met the conditions, if we have prayed sincerely from a heart fully surrendered to His will, then we can know this: Our God is able to heal. He has power enough. He loves us enough. And He *will* heal us—*if* He sees it is best for all concerned!

Isn't that enough? Can't we leave it with Him? Hasn't Calvary proven that we can trust Him?

Listen, friend. When we look long and earnestly at the cross of Calvary, when we see ourselves as we really are, and see what sinners we are, how we have crucified our Lord, how we have treated the One who loved us enough to die for us—physical healing won't seem so important. We will feel that if only our sins can be forgiven, if only the separation between us and our Saviour can be healed, nothing else really matters!

And that separation *can* be healed. It can be healed just now—without a moment's delay.

But don't be surprised if then, with every sin forgiven, you hear the words, "Get up and walk." Because the Saviour loves to speak those words. That's just the way He is!

Prescription for Tired Candles

The hero of Carmel lay down outside the city gate to sleep. He was tired, terribly tired, but happy. He had seen great things that day. God had been with him. God was with him now. He had no need to fear. He didn't need to hide anymore. Everything was going to be all right. As he dropped off to sleep, he was comforted by the sound of the driving rain that avalanched from the heavens as if trying to make up for the three and a half years of drought.

If Elijah had not been so tired, he would have happily reviewed the dramatic story that now appeared to have a happy ending. Israel had turned from the worship of the true God to the worship of Baal, a god of nature. Influenced by the wicked queen Jezebel and her four hundred and fifty false prophets, the people had decided that Baal, that pagan god of the sky, was responsible for the dew and the rain, for the blessings of nature that made their land a place of beauty. God had pleaded. He had sent His prophets. But Israel had turned a deaf ear. Now He must send a severe judgment.

So three and a half years ago God had sent Elijah to King Ahab with a weather forecast. No rain. At first the prediction was ridiculed. But as the land turned brown and streams ceased to flow, Ahab joined his queen and her prophets in hatred of the one who had brought the message and in seeking his life. God had miraculously protected him and fed him during his years of hiding. And then once again, at God's direction, Elijah stood in the presence of the king, who both hated and feared him.

Elijah demanded that the king and the prophets of Baal and all Israel, meet him atop Mount Carmel. It must be demonstrated, once and for all, who was the true God. At Elijah's direction the prophets of Baal had placed a sacrifice on their altar. Then for frantic hour after frantic hour they pleaded with Baal to send fire to consume it. But nothing happened. When finally they gave up and retired from the contest, Elijah repaired the altar of the Lord, placed a sacrifice upon it, and prayed a simple prayer. No sooner was his prayer ended than flames of fire, like brilliant flashes of lightning, descended from heaven, consuming not only the sacrifice but the stones of the altar as well!

What a moment! The king was awed. The people cried out with one voice, "The Lord, He is the God! the Lord, He is the God!" The prophets of Baal were destroyed. And God sent rain—such a rain that Ahab could not see to find his way down the mountain. So the humble prophet ran ahead of his chariot and guided him to the gate of the city.

Surely, thought Elijah, this was the beginning of a great reformation in Israel. The people had turned to the worship of the true God. The king had been profoundly impressed. The false prophets were gone. Surely the wicked Jezebel, when she heard what had happened, would be convinced that she could not win in her war against God. At least her strong influence over the king would be broken. No wonder Elijah could sleep peacefully and soundly.

But it was not to be. A messenger touched the tired prophet and awakened him. Jezebel, said the messenger, had vowed that by that hour tomorrow Elijah would be as dead as the false prophets!

It was too much! Evidently the reformation wasn't going to be so easy. Evidently the fury of Jezebel had not lessened. Evidently he was still to be a hunted fugitive. Exhausted as he was, awakened from a sound sleep, the disappointment hit him like a thunderbolt. Forgetting how God had worked for him in the past, Elijah ran for his life. He ran on and on until he found himself alone in a dreary, desolate waste. He sat down under a juniper tree to rest.

Elijah's candle was burning low—so low that now he didn't care if the flame did go out. He told God it was enough—and prayed that he might die. And then, utterly exhausted, he fell asleep.

Elijah should not have fled. He should not have permitted his faith to waver. The God who protected him as he stood alone on Carmel in the presence of those who would gladly have torn him in pieces if they had the opportunity—the God who protected him then could surely protect him from the wrath of one wicked woman. And if Elijah had kept a firm hold on his God, divine judgment would have fallen upon Jezebel. The king and the people would have been still more deeply impressed, and the reformation in Israel would have been greatly strengthened.

All this is true. But did God awaken Elijah and scold him for running away? No. God loved His faithful servant as much now as when he had stood firm as a rock. He let the tired man sleep. For sleep, not scolding, was what he needed now.

You see, God understood what Elijah had been through. He understood the limits of the human body and mind. Elijah had had a very hard day. For one thing, he had not eaten. The emotional strain had been tremendous. He had had to watch the false prophets every moment to see that by some trickery they did not succeed in lighting a fire on their altar. He had stood all day in the presence of those who desired to take his life. And then there was the physical strain of running before Ahab's chariot.

God knew that a reaction such as frequently follows high faith and glorious success was pressing upon Elijah. God knew, as we should know, that an emotional high is often followed by a corresponding letdown. Never has any man been involved in a more dramatic confrontation than was Elijah that day. No wonder he was exhausted. And no wonder that in his utter exhaustion he was seized by depression!

But watch how God treats exhaustion. Watch how He treats depression. First He lets him sleep. Then He sends an angel with food. Then He lets him sleep again. A second time the angel is sent to him. He touches the exhausted man and says ten-

derly, "Arise and eat; because the journey is too great for thee."
Elijah rose and ate, and in the strength of that food he was able
to walk forty days and forty nights to Horeb, the mount of God!

It was only then that God, kindly and gently, had a little talk
with Elijah about forsaking his post!

Sleep. Good food. Exercise. These are the remedies, these are
God's prescription for exhaustion and the depression that so often accompanies it.

But there is something else. We have missed the most important factor in bringing on Elijah's depression. True, he was exhausted physically and mentally and emotionally. But he was
not depressed until he let his faith slip, until he lost his hold on
God. Then he had reason to be depressed, for he was separated
from his God. No wonder he wanted to let his candle burn out—
clear out!

There is nothing, absolutely nothing, that makes you so tired
as *guilt*—as the knowledge that you are separated from your
God. And there is nothing, absolutely nothing, that will so renew your strength and your spirits, so set the heart to singing,
as the knowledge of forgiveness, the knowledge that the separation has been healed!

"Come unto Me," says the Saviour, "and I will give you rest."

Remember those words, that invitation, next time you feel
like a tired candle about to burn out. It's a prescription that
never fails!

Remember those words, that incredible opportunity next
time you sit with the broken pieces of your life about you on the
floor, too tired to pick them up. You don't have to sit and stare
at them in depression and remorse. There's a better way!

Forgiveness. Rest. And new strength—a brightly burning
flame of courage and faith and hope. All these await you at the
foot of an old-fashioned, splintery cross. But you'll never find
them anywhere else!

Tired—Ready to Break!

A book popular in the bookstores some years ago bore the title *How Never to Be Tired*. It had a phenomenal sale, because there are so many millions of tired people in the world.

And I have discovered, in meeting appointments across the country, that if I announce that I will speak about how never to be tired I don't need Madison Avenue publicity to get a crowd. Everybody is tired.

Tired—ready to break! And only one rope!

Every man, I say, begins life with a certain reserve of vital force, vital energy. Once it is gone, it cannot be replaced.

Many people use up this vitality, attempt to restore it from superficial supplies, and are tricked into thinking the loss has been made up by rest. On the contrary, every withdrawal of the deeper reserves of vital force leaves its scar. Somewhere the defenses are wearing thin. The body is only as strong as its weakest part. And someday, like the rope at the Portuguese monastery, it will break!

I am aware that men and women today are caught in the grip of tense nerves, the whirl of social commitments, the urge to meet the claims of custom, a chain of never-ending pressures that seem quite beyond their control. Anxiety and stress are in the air we breathe!

But millions keep themselves awake, keep themselves going, and try to solve their endlessly growing problems—with a streamlined pill. They ignore nature's red light and career blindly on.

159

Fatigue, you see, is nature's warning that vital energy is being exhausted. But men and women ignore the warning, put a penny in the fuse box by indulging in another cup of coffee, another cigarette, another pill—and carry on. And every penny in the fuse box teaches the nervous system to lie!

Tired—ready to break! Is it not time to ask, What makes a man tired?

Of course the suggestion that it is possible *never* to be tired obviously needs qualification. For there is a natural and normal weariness that comes from physical labor—a weariness that is quickly balanced by a good night's sleep. But there is also a tiredness that is not so replaced—a fatigue that dips into the reserves of vital force. This is the tiredness that concerns us. This is the tiredness that ought not to be.

What is it, then, that makes a man chronically tired? What is it that makes a man wish he could just stop like a run-down clock? Ever feel like that? What is it that makes some people even look longingly toward the future life as a time for endless, undisturbed rest?

My Bible doesn't picture the future life as a time of perpetual idleness. And I don't believe yours does either. Listen to this: "They that wait upon the Lord shall renew their strength; they shall mount up with wings as eagles; they shall run, and not be weary; and they shall walk, and not faint." Isaiah 40:31.

Tell me. Which would you rather have? Rest? Or renewed strength? Rest? Or new energy?

I have discovered that some scriptures have more than one application. Here we have a picture of the future life. But isn't it true that, even in this life, those who *run* are not so weary, that those who *walk* are not so faint?

Someone says, "Pastor Vandeman, I'm tired. Are you going to tell me that the way to get rested is to get out there and walk or run?"

That's what the walkers and the joggers will tell you. It's those who run, who jog, who walk—and do it regularly—that don't tire so easily. *Too much resting actually makes you tired.* Too much rest adds up to a cumulative fatigue, a chronic fatigue.

You see, you were never meant for inactivity. Everything in God's universe is in constant motion. The laws of nature, the laws of physics, the laws of space, are laws of action.

Stars and suns speed perpetually in their orbits. The earth revolves while it circles the sun. Rivers move toward the sea. The sea breaks against its shores. The sap flows in the trunks of the trees. The leaves appear. The blossoms bud. The grass springs up. The flowers unfold in all their delicate beauty.

Everything in the universe is active, vibrant, alive. Even the atoms are in constant motion, deep inside their prisons of wood or steel. Should man be idle? Should he covet a state of suspended activity that makes the blood flow sluggishly through his veins and causes his muscles to decrease in size and strength?

Inactivity makes you tired. A friend of mine told her experience of being in the hospital with scarlet fever when she was a teenager. She saw how weak the other patients were after being in bed for three weeks, and she determined it wouldn't happen to her. So every night, after lights were dimmed, she stood up on her bed and did some mild exercises. When she was given permission to get up for the first time, after three weeks, she slipped out of bed and played a game of ping pong with scarcely a sign of fatigue—much to the consternation of her doctor!

Well, I wouldn't recommend that you try her plan. It might be risky business. But it does make a point. *Lack of exercise makes you tired.*

And *drugs make you tired*—the ones you take to stimulate, to keep you going, to make you carry on when you ought to stop. Drugs such as caffeine in coffee and tea and cola drinks. And, of course, the pep pills.

Someone says, "But Pastor Vandeman, almost everyone uses one or more of these."

Yes. But it has been demonstrated sufficiently, I believe, that stimulants, sooner or later, will betray you. For there is always a reaction. Excitement is followed by depression. The nervous system, unduly excited, borrows power from the vital reserves. This temporary invigoration is followed by depression. Just in proportion as these stimulants temporarily invigorate, so there is a corresponding letdown.

These pep pills may look innocent enough. They may make you feel like a miracle—at first. But sooner or later these chemical crutches will trip you up. And, of course, with many of them, even coffeee, there is the danger of habit formation and even a form of addiction.

Coffee addiction? Cola addiction? Pep pills? Something to think about!

But you say, "I just have to have a stimulant. I have to have the extra pep. I just couldn't carry on."

Yes. But did you know that there are effective stimulants that have no depressing aftereffects? Of course, you won't find them on the drugstore shelves.

For instance, a hot shower in the morning—followed by *all cold*.

Some time ago I was meeting a series of appointments in one of the cities of the East, and I spoke one night on this subject, giving a little buildup for the cold shower. The next night I was handed this note:

"Dear Pastor Vandeman: This morning my husband said, 'If you hear a scream and see something blue running around, it will just be me. I'm going to take one of those cold showers.' Well, he did, and I haven't been able to do a thing with him all day. I'll have to take them too so I can manage him. I'm glad you stopped when you did."

Evidently I forgot to suggest a warm shower first!

Yes, if you want a stimulant, try a brief cold shower. And then, take your choice. Jogging, cycling, walking. They're the best. Or work in the garden, exercise in the open air. Whatever you wish. They're all yours—free—every one of them a stimulant, with no side effects. Guaranteed to take the cobwebs out of your mind—and the drag out of your step. No side effects, did I say? Well, maybe some sore muscles—at first.

Now is it possible that *a faulty diet can make you tired?*

Or put it another way. Does a healthful diet result in a lessening of fatigue? I believe it does. But more about that later. I'll be telling you about a people almost wholly free from fatigue—and what they eat.

Now we turn to the mind. *Depression makes you tired.* Probably more fatigue has resulted from depression than from any other cause. And *grief makes you tired. Anxiety makes you tired. Discontent, distrust, worry, fear, pain, home troubles*—all these tend to break down the life forces and invite not only fatigue but also disease and death.

On the other hand the contagion of courage, hope, and faith tends to promote healing and prolong life. The wise man said, "A merry heart doeth good like a medicine." Proverbs 17:22.

It is no surprise that *anger makes you tired,* that *hate makes you tired.* But *love renews. Love rejuvenates. Love heals.* And the whole body feels the touch of new life. Said a writer in whom I have confidence:

"The love which Christ diffuses through the whole being is a vitalizing power. Every vital part—the brain, the heart, the nerves—it touches with healing. By it the highest energies of the being are roused to activity. It frees the soul from the guilt and sorrow, the anxiety and care, that crush the life forces. With it come serenity and composure. It implants in the soul joy that nothing earthly can destroy."

Jesus said, "Thou shalt love thy neighbor as thyself." Could it be that those words are not so much a command as a prescription? Could it be that it is *love—or perish?*

Yes, *guilt makes you tired.* Guilt crushes the life forces. It unbalances the mind. Many a mind has been goaded to madness by the repetitious, trip-hammer accusing of the conscience. Guilt, if ignored too long, will poison the springs of life. Guilt can be lethal.

I am aware that Sigmund Freud, despite his pioneering of the mental sciences, once declared that God was guilty of a careless piece of work when He made the conscience. He saw everywhere the ravaging effects of guilt, you see, and he didn't understand. He tried to heal the fever by throwing away the thermometer. And so many a follower of Freud has tried to heal guilt by ignoring the conscience, making the conscience a scapegoat for man's sickness.

But guilt is not so easily dismissed. Conscience is not so easily quieted. Inner conflict results.

Guilt makes you tired, I say. But the Saviour says, "Neither do I condemn thee: go, and sin no more." And that changes it all.

Rest! Who doesn't need it in an hour like this? And it can be yours. Said our Lord, "Come unto me, all ye that labor and are heavy-laden, and I will give you rest. Take my yoke upon you, and learn of me; for I am meek and lowly in heart: and ye shall find rest unto your souls. For my yoke is easy, and my burden is light." Matthew 11:28-30.

Those words, friend, I sincerely believe, are a prescription that will touch and change every physical, mental, and spiritual problem known to man. They may sound too simple to work. But they have never failed.

You say, "Pastor Vandeman, I want that rest, that peace of mind, more than anything in the world. How can it be mine?"

It is not difficult or profound. It is within every man's reach. Surrender every tension. Remove every barrier. And let the Saviour heal.

And He will. You can find rest—even in a world like this. Through the forgiving, cleansing, healing power of Christ it is possible to live in a fortress of perfect peace. You can lay your guilt and your selfishness and your fear and everything that wearies the mind—you can lay it all at the foot of the cross and *never take it up again!*

What Faith Healers Don't Tell You

The story has burned across the gospel pages for nineteen centuries and more—the story of the woman who tremblingly, hesitatingly, reached out to touch the seamless robe of the Son of God.

Could it be that the Healer still is near enough that we moderns can touch His garment too—and live? What is the truth about divine healing?

When science has gone as far as it can, when all human help has failed, when we have followed one promise after another only to be disappointed—we remember the woman who touched His garment. And hope springs up that disease, and even death, may now, as then, be pushed back by the intervening hand of a great God.

It may have been a superstitious faith that she exercised that day. But it was faith nonetheless. Weak, timorous, maybe even theologically inaccurate. But it was the kind of faith that the Saviour delights to honor, even today.

Did you know that there are almost unbelievable promises in the Word of God about how and when and under what circumstances God will redeploy His own laws, invade the human personality if invited, change the course of nature if necessary—and heal? Promises like this: "Bless the Lord, . . . who forgiveth all thine iniquities; who healeth all thy diseases." Psalm 103: 2, 3. And this: "Pray one for another, that ye may be healed." James 5:16.

God does heal. There is no question about that. Jesus, while on earth, spent more time in healing than in preaching. Restoring men was His delight. And you can be assured that God desires to exercise His healing power today just as He did then.

Remember that God is not the originator of disease, suffering, and death. But He *is* the Author of laws that when violated bring trouble and pain. These bodies of ours are very obedient to the laws of cause and effect. And somewhere, sometime, somehow, we have to learn the truth that "whatsoever a man soweth, that shall he also reap." Galatians 6:7.

This truth works with mathematical precision. It works every time. But God lets us experiment if we must. He does not force the will.

For instance, our prisons and hospitals are filled with evidence of the effects of alcohol. But God does not knock the bottle out of a man's hand. Medical science now knows that smoking is linked with lung cancer. But God does not have an angel standing by to blow out the match. Any thinking man knows that overeating may contribute to a heart attack. But God does not push him back from the table when he has had enough. The time may come when a nurse will have to mark his menu. But God never does.

God does not force the will of man. But neither does He leave it without direction. He places the facts before us. If we choose to disobey, we choose also the consequences of disobedience.

I ask you, Would it be for man's best interest if God should, whenever requested, remove the illness that a man may have brought upon himself? If God should heal promiscuously, giving men new energies to burn out in continued disregard of the laws of health, would it be for their best good?

You see, God's plan for the restoration of man includes more than healing. It includes teaching him how to live. The Son of God traveled a long ladder down to where man was. But the ladder was intended to be traveled both ways. Jesus came not only to reach but also to lift. Never was His healing separated from His teaching.

You remember the man at the pool of Bethesda. Jesus said to him, "Take up thy bed, and walk." But a little later, in the temple, He said to him, "Sin no more, lest a worse thing come unto thee." John 5:8, 14.

Now it is our privilege to pray for healing, even if we have had something to do with bringing about the emergency. We are actually invited to pray for the healing we need; but we are also instructed to fulfill certain conditions and make certain adjustments in our living. I have repeatedly seen God honor His Word at the conclusion of reading and acting upon such words as these: "Is one of you ill? He should send for the elders of the congregation to pray over him and anoint him with oil in the name of the Lord. The prayer offered in faith will save the sick man, the Lord will raise him from his bed, and any sins he may have committed will be forgiven." James 5:14, 15, NEB.

When that plan is carefully and sincerely followed, when your desire is placed before God not in dictation or demand, but with a concentration of faith, in the strength of simple, un-adorned, relaxed believing, an answer always comes.

The answer may not come in just the way you expect. Some-times God heals instantly, sometimes gradually. And no thoughtful man would conclude that it is less an act of God to restore and heal over a longer period of time, permitting us to cooperate with Him in the healing process, than to heal in a more spectacular way. For it is *not the time element alone that makes healing divine.*

True, it requires nothing less than creative power to speak life to a decaying body. But did it ever occur to you that the same creative power revealed in the miracles of Jesus is con-tinuously at work in man's behalf? The creative power of God works through the agencies of nature, hour by hour, to sustain and restore us. Through the agencies of radiant sunlight, fresh air, cooling water, adequate rest, and pure food God lets down a ladder for our healing. And when we recover from illness, it is God who restores us.

God heals—sometimes instantly, sometimes gradually. Then sometimes God, who sees the future, as we do not, does not heal at all. He simply answers, No. But always remember—God is too wise to make a mistake and too good to be unkind.

You see, you might demand healing from God. And God

might give it. I am told that on one occasion a mother beat the air with her fists. She challenged God to heal her dying child. The child lived. But that unwise mother lived to see the day when that son was executed as a criminal.

All faith must be fitted around the final will of God. If Jesus needed to say, "Thy will be done," how much more do we need to say it! His will, we can always know, is for our best good. And in the end, as enlightened eyes look back upon difficult experiences, there will come from lips once bitter and critical the heartfelt words, "I see now. I wouldn't have had it any other way."

Yes, God still heals. He has made some striking promises about divine healing—promises that He honors again and again, wherever there is faith and a willingness to cooperate with the conditions that He has specified. Yet keep in mind that there is a counterfeit for every genuine doctrine, for every genuine gift of God.

God has said that miracles would be brought to their lowest abuse in the last days of world history. His Word tells us that before Christ's second coming counterfeit miracles will be performed in the name of religion—even in the name of Christ.

Remember the words of Jesus in Matthew 7, where He looked ahead to the judgment day and described the astonishment of certain miracle-working Christians when He would say, "I never knew you"? Listen:

"Not everyone who calls me 'Lord, Lord' will enter the kingdom of heaven, but only those who do the will of my heavenly Father. When that day comes, many will say to me, 'Lord, Lord, did we not prophesy in your name, cast out devils in your name, and in your name perform many miracles?' Then I will tell them to their face, 'I never knew you; out of my sight, you and your wicked ways!' " Matthew 7:21-23, NEB.

"What did He mean?" you ask. And you say, "Surely the devil would not bring into the lives of people such a wholesome benefit as healing, would he?"

Yes, evidently many will be healed by a power other than Christ's. And Christ—in whose name they are healed—will have nothing to do with it. Therein lies the subtle deception. "For there shall arise false Christs, and false prophets, and shall show great signs and wonders; insomuch that, if it were possible, they shall deceive the very elect." Matthew 24:24.

Now I would not judge the motives of any man or any group of men who claim the gift of healing. I know that many are sincere. But God will reveal to every man sufficient information to discern the true from the counterfeit. I do know that no people in all the history of this world have been called to face such deception as we.

Not all miracles, you see, are from God. Two forces are operating in this world. And only the man or the woman who takes time and sincere effort to understand the Word of God, who has an "It is written" as the basis for his action—only such individuals are safe from deception.

Never has the world been more in need of healing. And never have the healing lines been longer. There are the faith healers. There are the mass hypnotic healers. There are the trance healers, and the spirit healers.

Evidently there is need for a sharp distinction between true divine healing and the counterfeit. The two stand side by side. *Both are supernatural.* True, God honors genuine faith wherever He finds it. But the apostle Paul tells us that "Satan himself is transformed into an angel of light." 2 Corinthians 11:14. And Revelation 16:14 makes it clear that the spirits of demons in the last days will work miracles—not tricks. "For they are the spirits of devils, working miracles."

The man who accepts all that is miraculous as coming from God soon finds himself in a strange dilemma. For there are undoubted miracles in and out of the church. There are miracles all through the cults. There are miracles in spiritism. There are miracles even in the voodoo rites of Haiti. But here is the point. Shall he accept the *teaching* because of the *miracle?* What sort of faith would be his if he did?

Remember that to turn aside from Scripture is to walk on ice that is treacherously thin. For miracles can never take the place of knowing and following the will of God. It is a dangerous thing to make a miracle the price of your soul!

"How then can I distinguish between true and false healing?" you ask.

I sincerely believe that there are earmarks, questions, and contrasts that, if kept in mind, will keep you from serious deception on this vital point.

Does the healer *demand* healing from God? Or does he teach his people to say, "Thy will be done"?

Does he exalt Christ as the Great Physician? Or does he make God only a sort of publicity agent to further his own personal fame?

Does he stay close to Scripture? If not, the words of Isaiah apply: "To the law and to the testimony: if they speak not according to this word, it is because there is no light in them." Isaiah 8:20.

Does the healer tell those who come to be healed that their illness may be the result of their own disobedience to nature's laws? Does he teach them how to cooperate with those laws in the future?

Does the healer tell his people about the healing power of *sunlight* as it is allowed to shower its radiant energy over body and soul?

Does he tell them of the healing potential of ordinary *water*— skillfully, scientifically, generously used, inside and out? Does he tell them about the relaxing effects of simply watching water in motion—a waterfall, or even a fountain in the backyard? There is something about watching water in action that seems to unwind nerves, take the kinks out of muscles, and remove strain from the heart.

Does he tell men and women how to take a tip from their heart, and *rest* between the beats?

Does he tell them about pure, fresh *air*, God's air-conditioning system for body and mind? Air means oxygen. And oxygen means life. Reduce a man's supply of oxygen and the higher centers of his brain are affected first. A man's judgment and memory are so impaired that even ordinary questions are answered stupidly. Reason enough for getting plenty of fresh air?

Does the healer explain what happens to a man when he neglects *exercise*? Does he explain that we must keep our nerves in balance—that unless we balance mental activity with physical exercise, sooner or later the mainspring is going to snap? A good brisk walk every day is cheaper and safer and far more interesting than a nervous breakdown.

And does the healer say a word about *diet*—those fruits, grains, nuts, and vegetables that the Creator chose for the human race? Does he tell his people that such a diet, when it is followed with wisdom and simplicity, will be a giant step toward radiant health? Does he tell them that the body is the temple of God? Remember? Does he ever read them the words of Paul—words so forthright I almost hesitate to read them? "If any man defile the temple of God, him shall God destroy." 1 Corinthians 3:17. Does he teach them the underlying principle to be followed in eating and drinking? "Whether therefore ye eat, or drink, or whatsoever ye do, do all to the glory of God." 1 Corinthians 10:31.

Could it be that what we eat or drink has more to do with the health of the soul than we have realized? Evidently.

This brings us to the fundamental difference between true and false healing. One deals only with the momentary need of the body. The other, along with healing, teaches men how to live in harmony with the laws of the Creator. One promises life in obedience—the other in disobedience. In counterfeit healing there is no recognition of the part sin may have played in producing illness, and no turning away from it. But the Saviour says to every man, "Go, and sin no more."

The healing of the body. The healing of the soul. And who can say which is the greater miracle?

"How thankful I am that God not only said to Roy Slaybaugh, 'Take up your bed and walk,' but that He also said to me, 'Your sins are forgiven.' "

These were the words of Berkley Jones, once a desperate criminal, his picture in every guard tower, with orders to shoot to kill if he should step out of bounds.

Berkley Jones, with his brother, had escaped from prison with the help of a pistol. They were racing at eighty-five miles an hour around a curve on a narrow country road when they collided with Roy Slaybaugh—and left him for dead.

But God miraculously and instantaneously healed the torn and battered body—even to restoring a missing eye, a mangled ear, and a broken jaw. Medical records authenticate this unusual healing.

After repeated attempts, Roy Slaybaugh gained permission to visit Berkley and his brother in the Oregon State Penitentiary. A deep friendship sprang up. Both boys gave their hearts to Christ. Both were paroled. Berkley attended a Christian college and for years faithfully witnessed for his Lord in working for youth.

Talking with Berkley Jones, I looked into the face of one redeemed by a miracle as great as the re-creation of a torn, broken body. Here was a re-created soul. Imagine him—once a desperate criminal, his picture in every guardhouse—imagine him talking to me like this, as he described his first meeting with the man he had so greatly wronged:

"Here was the man I had seen practically dead beside the road the day I hit him. Now I saw how God had healed him. And then to know that this man could forgive me the terrible wrong I had done to him. For the first time I saw what forgiveness meant. It was that which led me to Christ."

And then he concluded, "How thankful I am that God not only said to Roy Slaybaugh, 'Take up your bed and walk,' but that He also said to me, 'Your sins are forgiven.' "

Yes, who can tell which is the greater miracle? Both require the creative power of God. But while one restores life here, the other means life eternal.

Friend, please know that God will hear your sincere prayer for the healing of the body. But the ears of a loving heavenly Father are even more eager to hear the prayer, "Lord, be merciful to me, a sinner." God never says No, or even Wait, to this request!

The Winds of the Witches

Witches' winds, they call them. The *foehn* (fān) of Austria and Switzerland, the Mediterranean *sirocco*, and the *mistral* of France. The *hamsin* of Israel. The *chinook* of the Rocky Mountains. And the *Santa Ana* of southern California.

There seems to be something mysterious about these winds, something sinister. Are they the revengeful punishment meted out by an environment we have betrayed—or by an angry God? Is there really any witchcraft?

Or is there a simple, fascinating, and significant explanation?

They have certain distinct characteristics—these mysterious winds, these *foehn* winds. They occur on the leeward slope of a mountain range. The air, at first, is a cold mass. But it warms as it comes down the mountain, and appears finally as a hot, dry wind.

The Santa Ana, in southern California, blows down through the Cajon Pass, drying the hills to a flash point. The humidity is low, and this incendiary dryness invariably means fire. You see smoke back in the canyons and hear sirens in the night. The wind may gust to a hundred miles an hour!

It was the Santa Ana that caused Malibu to burn as it did in 1956, and Bel Air in 1961, and Santa Barbara in 1964 and again in 1977. The wind seems to be a harbinger of catastrophe. And some, when the wind and the flames come too close, envision Los Angeles itself coming to its end in flames fanned by the Santa Ana!

But these *foehn* winds are more than the threat of fire. They affect people too. In Switzerland the suicide rate goes up during the *foehn*. In some Swiss courts the wind is considered a mitigating circumstance for crime. It is said that surgeons watch the winds, because blood does not clot normally during a *foehn*.

Whenever these strange winds blow, doctors hear about headaches and nausea and allergies and nervousness and depression. Moods are often profoundly affected. North Africans say that when the *sirocco* blows off the Sahara, it depresses people to the point of suicide.

To put it simply, these winds sometimes make people very unhappy!

But why? Is it really mystery or magic—or witchcraft?

The common factor in all these winds is the *ion*. The *ion* is a molecule that has become electrically charged as a result of gaining or losing an electron. And of course this is happening all the time. The ions become negatively charged or positively charged, depending on the prevailing conditions.

The earth, you see, is always negatively charged. So when the air is clean and moist—as it is in forests, near lakes and streams, or on mountains—the positive ions that are generated by collisions of water droplets are quickly absorbed into the ground. This leaves the atmosphere charged with negative ions, which is the ideal situation.

Do you see now why health spas are always located near waterfalls or seashores or forests or on mountains—and also why these places are popular vacation choices? You feel better on vacation not simply because of the beautiful scenery, or because you're not working, but because of the air you breathe.

But what happens when these hot, dry winds blow? Positive ions are generated. And they can't be neutralized, because there is no moisture for the earth to absorb. So these winds are saturated with high concentrations of positive ions.

An Israeli physicist has discovered that this high concentration of positive ions exists not only during the winds, but for ten or twelve hours preceding them.

Something similar happens before a thunderstorm. Have you ever noticed that you feel depressed when a storm is building up, but that when it breaks you feel better? That's because a thundercloud, as it moves, sweeps away the negative ions under it, leaving the air positively charged. But when the storm breaks and the lightning takes over, large numbers of negative ions are discharged into the air. The atmosphere is normal again.

The research of the past twenty years all points to this—that positive ions make people sick, and that negative ions enhance health. In fact, the effect of large concentrations of negative ions is actually exhilarating.

Dr. Albert Krueger, a microbiologist and experimental pathologist at the University of California at Berkeley, discovered that even a small concentration of negative ions could kill airborne bacteria that cause colds and flu and other respiratory problems. Dr. Krueger, along with others, has shown that negative ions stimulate the cells in the body that help us to resist disease.

A Philadelpia physician demonstrated that his burn patients suffered much less pain—and recovered more quickly—when negative-ion generators were placed in their rooms. And there was less danger of infection, with not so much scarring.

Dr. Krueger has found evidence that an excess of positive ions causes overproduction of the stress hormone serotonin in mammals. And serotonin is definitely associated with sudden changes in mood. When too much of it is secreted into the bloodstream, it causes anxiety, insomnia, and migraine headaches. People who suffer acutely from the effects of the dry winds actually have an average increase of 1000 percent in the serotonin level of their blood.

On the other hand, Dr. Krueger proved that the tranquilizing effect of negative ions is because the amount of serotonin in the midbrain is reduced.

But now why all this? Why is it that positive ions make people feel worse and negative ions make them feel better? Here's the key. Dr. Krueger and the Russian scientist D. A. Lapitsky both tell us that *without the presence of negative ions we cannot absorb the oxygen essential to life.*

Evidently human beings are actually "bio-electric" creatures designed to function best at certain levels of air eletricity. It isn't witchcraft in the hot, dry winds. It's a simple problem of the level of electricity, the kind of electricity, in the air we breathe.

So what can we do about it? Think it through. There are huge concentrations of positive ions, the damaging ones, in automobiles, in airplanes, in the buildings in which we work. Congested cities fairly fester with massive concentrations of positive ions. We are paving over our earth with asphalt and concrete, and pollutants from cars and other sources are trapped in our concrete canyons. Technology is distorting the electrical charge of the air we breathe. And we may be almost strangling ourselves without knowing it!

Oxygen. Pure, fresh air. Meant to electrify our bodies. Meant to give us energy. Meant to invigorate. Without it not a cell of our bodies can live. Without it we cannot have good blood. Without it we cannot have a good circulation. Without it the brain cannot function properly. And that's getting pretty close home!

Brain cells that are deprived of sufficient oxygen simply do not function efficiently. That means that we aren't alert. That means that our powers of reason begin to fade. A man doesn't have to be deprived of oxygen very long until he begins to give stupid answers to the questions asked him.

Some years ago a French investigator was interested in high altitude flying and arranged for three balloonists to make an ascent. They had ballast, they had ropes, they had oxygen. But not oxygen enough for the entire flight, so they agreed to use it only when necessary.

All went well for a time. Then they began to notice that they had strange emotions they could not control. They would laugh or cry without reason. There was reason enough, of course. The oxygen was gone.

They knew something was wrong. They knew they should descend. The rope was there. The knife to cut the rope, thus releasing some of the hydrogen, was there. But the power to execute that simple act of cutting the rope was gone!

Three days later when the balloon finally landed several

hundred miles away, two of the three balloonists were dead. The other told the story.

And this little story tells us a lot. These men, deprived of adequate oxygen, still had good judgment. They knew what they ought to do. Their self-control, their emotional control, was already affected. But their willpower was gone completely!

Evidently willpower is the first to go. And of course if the lack of oxygen continues, self-control and good judgment will go too—likely in that order. But willpower goes first!

Does that ring some bells? Many a man has good judgment. And he may still have self-control. But his willpower is gone.

I have said it before, but please let me say it again— particularly at this point: this is the cry of thousands of alcoholics. No willpower. And a legion of smokers echo it. No willpower. It is the plaintive cry of millions of weight watchers who put off their weight watching until tomorrow. And the uncounted victims of temper and lust join in. No willpower. It is a cry of defeat that makes the heart of God weep!

Do you see now why smokers find it so hard to quit? No smoker gets adequate oxygen. No wonder his willpower is gone!

And what about the important decisions, the far-reaching decisions, that are made in smoke-filled rooms where the oxygen is so severely depleted that not much more than survival is possible? Is it any wonder that mistakes in judgment are made?

I say again, God lets us decide ourselves what our eternal destiny shall be. But what if we are deliberately impairing our decision-making powers? What if we are making ourselves incapable of wise decisions?

A nineteenth-century writer in whom I have great confidence, and one with an unusual grasp of the mental sciences, made this intriguing statement: "The brain nerves which communicate with the entire system are the only medium through which Heaven can communicate to man."

Think of it! The brain nerves—the only way God can communicate with us, with the mind, with the conscience! What if the brain nerves aren't getting enough oxygen? What if the brain is unable to discriminate between right and wrong?

Am I suggesting that our eternal destiny could actually depend upon how much oxygen we are getting? Yes, I am!

You see, if we don't get enough oxygen to keep the will and the conscience functioning properly, we may just coast along, partially stupefied, knowing what we ought to do, but helpless to cut the ropes of habit, the ropes of sin. And there's no greater tragedy than an anesthetized will!

No wonder Solomon said, "Guard your heart [your mind] more than any treasure." Proverbs 4:23, NEB.

Guard your mind, friend. You're going to need it. Beware of anything that dulls your mental powers. Alcohol does it. Tobacco does it. Overeating does it. Fatigue does it. A lack of oxygen does it.

So how shall we go about making sure that from this moment on we do get the fresh air, the oxygen, that is so vital to radiant health? Let's be practical.

1. Make your home, if you can, where the air is unpolluted. Country living is best.

2. Let the fresh air in. Let it blow through the house. Remember that indoor air could be hazardous to your health.

3. Learn to breathe right, if you don't already know. And if you do know, practice it. Use the abdominal muscles, use the diaphragm, in breathing. Breathe deeply.

4. Exercise. Don't overdo it. But don't neglect it. To neglect it is to take chances with your health, with your life, with your destiny.

And then I wouldn't want to close this chapter without making another application, a more directly spiritual one. It is this. Prayer is the breath of the soul, the oxygen of the soul. Just as we can't live physically without oxygen, so we can't live spiritually without prayer, without communication with our God. We neglect it at our peril!

It may be that the channel of communication is clogged, is blocked. Said the prophet Isaiah, "But your iniquities have made a separation between you and your God, and your sins have hid His face from you, so that He does not hear." Isaiah 59:2, NASB.

So if the channel is blocked, let's unblock it. How long would we tolerate a choked gas line on one of our cars?

Our biggest problem, our most serious problem, is not the hot, dry winds—the winds of the witches. There's no witchcraft involved in those winds.

Our greater concern should be the winds of temptation that bewitch us and threaten our will to cut the ropes of sin. Our greater concern should be to stay away from Satan's enchanted ground, because that's where the winds of temptation blow. That's where they sweep away our willpower and spoil our contact with Heaven and threaten our destiny!

We've been talking again about the law of cause and effect, about the law that says, "A man reaps what he sows." Galatians 6:7, NIV.

But here's a happy thought. Here's a positive note. Too often we forget that the law of cause and effect works both ways. It can work for us as well as against us.

We have learned the hard way that the consequences of extreme carelessness are not pleasant. And so we manage to avoid the worst. We go through life content with barely avoiding the headache, the allergy reaction, the heart attack. We go through day after day, month after weary month, breathing just enough fresh air to keep us from being stupid. When all the time we could set our course so that the law of cause and effect would work in our favor. When all the time the life-giving oxygen, the gift of our Creator, is all about us, free for the taking. When, beginning just now, we could experience the new, vibrant, radiant health we were intended to possess!

And there's no better place to begin than in the fresh air, with even before that a little time—decision-making time, destiny-producing time—on our knees!

Guilt Can Be Lethal

In the sixth century before Christ, so an ancient fable says, the Greek lyric poet Ibycus, on his way to the festival of music at Corinth, was attacked and killed by two robbers. But just as he was dying, he saw a flock of cranes flying overhead and called upon them to avenge his death. And the robbers heard him.

All Greece was shocked by the violent death of Ibycus, and the people urged the authorities to bring the offenders to punishment. But this seemed impossible, for there had been no witnesses to the crime.

A few days later, in Corinth, in a theater open to the sky, a huge audience sat spellbound. It so happened that the choristers were impersonating the Furies, as they were called, the goddesses of vengeance. And such a performance, considering the angry mood of the people, seemed uncannily appropriate. No one was aware that in that theater, on the top benches, sat the two murderers.

In solemn step the singers slowly advanced. They were clad in black robes and carried torches that blazed with flame. Their cheeks were pale as death, and in place of hair they wore crowns of writhing serpents. Their weird song of vengeance rose higher and higher until it paralyzed the hearts and chilled the blood of the hearers.

At that very moment a flock of cranes swept across the sky and passed low over the theater. Instantly, from those top benches, there was a cry of terror. "Look, comrade! Look! Yonder are the cranes of Ibycus!"

Every eye turned in the direction of that telltale cry of guilt. The murderers had informed against themselves. The atmosphere of vengeance, and the sudden appearance of those ill-omened cranes, to them the harbingers of swift revenge, had been too much for them.

And so the *cranes of Ibycus* have become synonymous with the truth that guilt will out.

Who of us does not identify in some way with this fable? Who of us, at some time, surprised by our own personal cranes of Ibycus, has not cried out in the darkened theater of the mind, "I am guilty!"

And you have only to open your eyes to see around you, even within the circle of family and friends and work associates, a huge crowd of wounded and distressed men and women who are crushed by hidden guilt. That guilt may be real or imagined, definite or vague, recognized or unrecognized. But it is there. There is even a sort of guilt at being alive—and it is more common than you think.

And guilt can be lethal to the human personality. There is nothing in this world so destructive to inner peace as the sense of guilt. In fact, one writer remarks that "guilt as virulent as in the days of the medieval torture chambers has put modern psychology in business."

Yes, the most persistent enemy of man's inner peace, the most difficult to eradicate, the one that refuses to be bypassed or ignored or explained away, is guilt. Guilt is what is bugging this generation.

Now who doesn't agree that guilt throws sand into the machinery of the mind? But what about the body? Wouldn't it be utterly inconceivable that guilt, so devastating to the mind, should not also work havoc with the physical health?

Actually, the concept that emotional states affect the body is comparatively new in medical thinking. But did you know that millenniums ago the Scriptures clearly stated it? Listen to these:

"A mind at ease is life and health, but passion makes man rot away." "Trouble wears away my strength, I age under outrages." "There is no health in my limbs, thanks to my sins."

Proverbs 14:30; Psalm 6:7; Psalm 38:3. All three texts from Moffatt's translation.

I never tire of reading the story of the man who was brought to Jesus on a stretcher. Jesus was teaching in a house, you recall, but it was impossible to get through the crowd; so the sick man's friends tore up the roof and let him down directly in front of the Healer. Tearing up the roof in those days, of course, was a relatively simple matter, and there is no record that the householder even protested.

Isn't it interesting that the Healer responded to all this urgency and determination and evident faith not by immediately healing the man, but rather by forgiving his sins? "Seeing their faith Jesus said to the man, 'Take heart, my son; your sins are forgiven.' " Matthew 9:2, NEB.

Forgiveness. Was that what he had come for? Wouldn't it be enlightening to know all the significant details that are not included in the brief Scripture account?

Could it be that the man's illness may have been a result of his sin? Could it be that forgiveness was what he really wanted—more than healing? Could it be that the divine Healer may have been watching the man's deep repentance—watching as his friends slowly made their way with their patient along the dusty roads—watching as he urged his friends to tear away the roof, anything that he might reach the Saviour?

"Take heart, my son; your sins are forgiven." See the stricken man lying there upon his stretcher now—relaxed, perfectly content, forgiven. Did physical healing even matter now? Or were the words of Jesus that followed—"take up your bed and walk"—just an extra bonus?

I think so. One thing is certain. Jesus understood the inseparable relationship of guilt and disease. And He demonstrated that guilt can be healed.

But guilt, to be healed, must first be recognized. And modern man would rather do anything than to recognize it. He tries to deny it, bypass it, ignore it, suppress it, explain it away.

But conscience has a memory like an elephant. It keeps coming back. And so man tries to heal guilt by discarding his conscience. He tries to heal the fever by throwing away the thermometer.

Let me put it this way. In a court of law a man tries to establish his innocence by proving either that he did not break the law or that there was no law to break.

The same thing goes on within the human personality. Conscience is the prosecuting attorney. Memory is the incriminating witness. But the mind of man either denies that he has broken the law—or protests that there was no law to break. The latter argument is supposed to throw the whole case out of court—except that guilt is not so easily quieted.

I need not tell you that the defense strategy of this generation is that there is no law to break.

If we have no standards, you see, there can be no violation of them. We took *sin* out of our vocabulary and thought that settled the matter. There was no such thing as sin, we were told. Sin was either bad form or something psychological. Listen to David Redding:

"Modern men have further established their innocence by abolishing the word 'sin' altogether." We dismiss sin, he says, "as a subnormal notion great-grandfather entertained. Sin to them is only a phantom that rattled the shutters of early Americana."

And he continues, "Making guilt inadmissable has made it all the more dangerous. Since it is undefined, sin now enjoys a reign of terror. We refuse to believe that there is anything to forgive."

But guilt, I say, will not be so easily quieted. The cranes of Ibycus keep flying over our heads.

For decades now we have been watching a gradual erosion of our moral values. The culture of the eighties tells us that these things don't matter. But down deep in our hearts we know that they do.

Many a man has discovered, by indelible experience, that if he knows a thing is wrong, it doesn't matter how many people, how many counselors, how many magazines, how many books, tell him it is right. Conscience must answer to God, not to public opinion. And conscience keeps remembering what God says about sin.

Listen to four short, crisp statements of Scripture:

"Sin is the transgression of the law." "The wages of sin is death." "All have sinned, and come short of the glory of God." "The heart is deceitful above all things, and desperately wicked." 1 John 3:4; Romans 6:23; Romans 3:23; Jeremiah 17:9.

That's what God says. But our modern, sophisticated pride makes it difficult to accept a Saviour. It's easier to accept therapy. It's easier to blame society—to blame our environment, our childhood, our chromosomes, or other people. Somebody in City Hall is responsible. Somebody in Washington. But not me.

But my guilt is never healed until it is recognized—until I place the blame on me. It is never healed until I come to the place where I say, "I am to blame. No one else is responsible. God help me!"

Only the guilty can be forgiven. A physician is useless to the man who says he is not sick. The Son of God came not "to call the righteous, but sinners to repentance." That's what He said. And the apostle Paul said, "Christ Jesus came into the world to save sinners; of whom I am chief."

It isn't easy to take the blame. How many apologies have come your way that canceled themselves out with qualifications and explanations and excuses that left them lifeless and meaningless? How many apologies like that have you made? And how many prayers?

Rosalind Rinker relates how she, with two other young missionaries in China, determined in their prayer group to make their prayers personal and conversational and honest. One day she decided that her prayer would be one of admission concerning her strong tendency to be "bossy"—to imagine that her ideas were superior to those of others and far more workable.

"Lord," she began, "if I have been—" She stopped, sensing she was giving herself a "leg to stand on," which she really didn't mean to do. She started over. "Dear Lord, I sometimes have a tendency to—" She stopped again. She knew that at that moment she was still not taking any personal responsibility for her actions and attitude. She started a third time—with determination. "Dear Lord Jesus, forgive me for always thinking my way is better, and for always wanting to 'boss' everything." She stopped, knowing she had finally revealed the truth without rationalizing.

Her friends picked up this fragment of conversational prayer. One of them said, "Thank You, Lord, for Ros's honesty." And the other prayed, "Yes, thank You. We have always known she was like this, but it sure helps us to hear her admit it."

When I first heard that story, I knew she was talking about me. For I must confess that I am sure there have been times when my family and friends would have been deeply relieved to hear me pray in a spirit like that, acknowledging that I too make mistakes and sometimes make others unhappy.

Fortunately, these imperfections of character, freely confessed, can be corrected by the grace of God. But the guilt that haunts the conscience, unbalances the mind, and damages the body often involves sins not so easily corrected, crime that cannot be undone.

A minister in his sermon told of a woman who had made restitution for some stolen ducks. And another woman said to him, "It is easy to make restitution about ducks. But I stole another woman's husband."

Yes, more may be involved than ducks. A man may be guilty of crime so serious that his hopelessness and despair cannot be described. He may be forever haunted by the irreversibility of what he has done. He may feel an extremity of blame that seems beyond the reach of forgiveness.

But it isn't, friend. God says, "Him that cometh to me I will in no wise cast out." And "if we confess our sins, he is faithful and just to forgive us our sins, and to cleanse us from all unrighteousness."

Abraham Lincoln, not long before his death, was asked how he would treat the defeated Southerners. And he replied, "As if they had never been away."

That's the way God forgives. That's the way He accepts us—as though we had never sinned.

Someone is saying, "Pastor Vandeman, this is all so wonderful. But doesn't guilt have to be punished?"

Yes, it does. That's what Calvary is all about. Sin had to be punished. But the Son of God bore our guilt. "He was wounded for our transgressions, he was bruised for our iniquities. . . . The Lord hath laid on him the iniquity of us all."

You say, "Does this mean that my sins—even mine—can be forgiven?"

Yes, even yours. Even mine.

A narrative from old Scotland tells of an elderly man who sat through the communion service, feeling too unworthy to partake. He sat there miserably, feeling he dare not participate in this memorial of his Lord's death.

And then he saw a teenage girl break down and pass the cup untasted. Suddenly his fears were gone, and he cried out to her in a loud whisper, "Take it, lassie! Take it! It's for sinners!"

And then he too reached out with eager hands to take it for himself.

Take it, friend! Take it! It's for sinners!

The Other Side of Grief

Grief—how that word haunts us. How can we be prepared to handle this trauma that comes one time or other to us all?

When the doctor arrived, he found Emma in a frightening state of despair. She was terribly agitated; no one could calm her. The woman rushed about her room, deaf to the pleas of her family. She threw herself on the bed and began shouting curses. The doctor managed to tell her that he had come to help.

But Emma jumped to her feet and shouted, "I don't need a doctor! I'm not ill! Give me back my daughter! My little girl."

Emma had just entered the dark, disordered world of grief. Those inside that world often wonder, "Will there ever be a way out?"

No one wants to be a good loser—especially when the loss is a loved one. But losses happen, tragic accidents claim their victims, divorce shears the deepest bonds, families are uprooted, cancer and heart disease strike the unsuspecting.

An extended family used to provide support during times of mourning. We had a large network of friends who saw us through the tears. But in our mobile world today, full of high-rise isolation and fragmented families, support is harder to come by. There are fewer shoulders to cry on.

The loss of a loved one usually brings on us dozens of overpowering emotions. At first, shock numbs all feeling. But then the pain begins to pierce. We sometimes lash out in anger, without knowing why. Friends find it hard to relate. Rapid mood swings send some mourners into isolation. As one man said, "There is a sort of invisible blanket between the world and me." Remaining alone and confused often brings on depression. Handling the simplest tasks becomes a tiresome burden.

Some feel trapped by unfocused fears and a vague sense of guilt. They ask, "Why did I survive?" And they wonder, "Am I somehow responsible for this terrible loss?" Frequently those experiencing grief feel that God has deserted them. They come seeking comfort and find a door slammed in their faces. They sometimes ask, "Why does God seem so absent in times of trouble?"

At times the hardest thing to bear is the "comfort" of those who come with good intentions. At the funeral someone says, "You know, death is just a door. Death really doesn't exist for a Christian." But oh, how it DOES exist at that moment. It DOES matter to you, who have just lost the dearest thing in life.

Others might try to comfort you by saying, "Your son is asleep with God." But you don't want your child with God. You desperately want him back. Friends drop in and praise you for bearing the loss so well. Such courage and faith are admirable. But your stolid exterior is just a mask. You're too numb or angry for tears and want to scream, "No, no, I'm not handling this well at all."

Then friends come with advice. "Just try to forget," they counsel, "and you'll get over it." But your greatest fear is that you *will* forget. You are anxiously trying to remember all you can. Because in the emotional turmoil of grief, even familiar memories grow hazy. Others tell you to keep busy, not to stop and think, it only makes it worse. But you are already straining to accomplish the simplest tasks. More to do only increases your disorientation.

Real comforters are hard to come by. Sometimes you feel like you must simply grieve alone. Misery may love company, but it certainly doesn't attract any.

I have not been without grief in my life. I've known the cutting edge of tragedy. No, I have not lost those nearest me—our losses have been in the extended family. Through tragic death we lost two fine young nephews. And others in the family, of course, have been laid to rest one by one through the years.

In and through all of this tragedy I have shared the God of all comfort with those remaining—that they nor I need not mourn alone because we know One who grieves with us. The prophet Isaiah describes Him as "a man of sorrows and acquainted with grief." Isaiah 53:3, NKJV.

This is the Christ, the One who cried out from the cross, "My God, my God, why have you forsaken me?" Mark 15:34.

That desperate cry takes in all our cries of grief—from Adam and Eve, wailing over the death of Abel, to today's Lebanese mother, weeping over a child slain by a terrorist bomb.

Jesus understands the despair of grief. And I believe He has also given us the resources to work through our grief and recover from its despair. We can take certain steps to prevent grief from hardening into bitterness. We can grow through our sorrow. We CAN reach the other side.

All of us have different capacities for dealing with loss, just as some bear physical pain better than others. Grief is never exactly the same in any two people. Much depends on the kind of relationship we had with the loved one who is gone.

But we all need to understand that grieving is a normal, healthy process. It is not an illness; it is not neurotic. Mourning is a way to get our lives back in focus again. The first step in healthy mourning is to express our feelings. Shock may keep us silent the first few days following a traumatic loss, but as the numbness wears off and emotions begin to flood in—we need an outlet. Find someone who will listen without judging, who will understand without trying to give a lot of advice.

In Bible times, people could express their grief very dramatically. They tore their garments, poured ashes over their heads, and put on sackcloth. Their weeping and wailing was accepted as a normal response to sorrow. Today we tend to emphasize composure and quiet mourning. But we still need a way to express the pain of loss.

When Mr. Kay received a telegram from the navy telling him his son was missing in action, he took the news stoically. Although Mr. Kay had always idolized his son, he never broke down or showed any visible emotion. Friends commented on how bravely he bore the tragedy.

But Mr. Kay, who had a very successful business, began making unwise and careless investments. He buried himself in books about warfare and became obsessed with finding out everything he could about the Civil War. He insisted that family members stay close by, but never shared his feelings with them. Mr. Kay became increasingly irritable and bitter. Finally his pent-up emotions brought on a serious illness.

Mr. Kay had not been able to deal with his grief directly. So it manifested itself in other problems. He badly needed to share the pain that was tying knots inside him. In His Sermon on the Mount, Jesus gave this beatitude: "Blessed are those who mourn, for they will be comforted." Matthew 5:4, NIV.

Mourning brings comfort. Those who refuse to face their loss and share their pain with others can't be adequately comforted. Now in this first step of talking it out, we can't expect to praise God for the tragedy. Some well-meaning people tell grieving friends, "Well, after all, it was God's will. It's all for the best."

But death and separation don't feel like the best at all. In the painful shock following a sudden loss, we see only darkness— we can't make out any stars in the black heavens. We feel that God isn't there, that He's abandoned us. And listen, those feelings are legitimate. Remember the heart-wrenching cry of Jesus on the cross: "Why, why have You forsaken Me?" Death and tragedy strike precisely because we live in a world that has cut itself off from God. Evil rules here. Death doesn't feel like God's will—of course not. Death is evil. Period.

Now, God *does* promise to work good out of evil. He hasn't abandoned us any more than He abandoned His suffering Son. God can turn bitterness into blessing.

But at first we can't see that. We can barely see at all. The world is shrouded in the gloom of our numb grief. And in the beginning, we don't have to see. It's OK to mourn the evil of death. It's OK to share our grief over the evil of separation.

After we have talked out our feelings, we can begin a period of adjustment. This may take many months. We have to adjust to a home where the loved one is missing. So many things remind us of the person who should be there. We walk down a familiar path and feel the hand that used to hold ours. In the late afternoon we still half-consciously listen for footsteps at the door. We wake in the night, reach across the bed, and find an empty pillow.

Adjustment means we must take care of life's details in a new way. We may have to assume new responsibilities. As much as possible, we need to make these adjustments one step at a time. During periods of stress it's best to simplify our lifestyle. The help of friends and neighbors can be vital during this time.

Madge was busily preparing to fly home to be with her mother. Several members of the family had been killed in a car crash. The terrible news came just as Madge, her husband, and children were preparing to move to a new state. The house was in chaos. Somehow Madge had to get ready for the funeral. She had to find the right clothes for everyone in all the boxes and suitcases. As she was walking around the house in a daze, aimlessly picking things up and putting them down, the doorbell rang.

It was a neighbor. "I've come to clean your shoes," he said. Madge didn't understand. So the neighbor explained, "When my father died, it took me hours to get the children's shoes cleaned and shined for the funeral. So that's what I've come to do for you." The neighbor settled himself on the kitchen floor and scraped and washed and shined all the shoes in the house. Watching him concentrate quietly on his task helped Madge pull her thoughts together and begin her own preparations. Later, when Madge returned from the laundry room, the neighbor was gone. But lined neatly against the wall stood all their shoes, spotless and gleaming.

Acts of kindness can make such a difference as we go through the difficult period of adjustment during mourning. When friends call and ask, "Is there anything I can do to help?" it is difficult for the bereaved to answer. Much better are offers to do specific tasks: "Let me take care of the children tonight," or, "Could I get your groceries this week?"

After adjusting to a loss, and after we have begun to carry on basic tasks again, we can begin the process of *renewal*. We can take a more active part in our healing as we redirect our emotions and energies into new channels. You might start by making a list of your personal assets. What gifts or abilities do you have that could be developed? Then write down a few short-term goals for yourself. How can you put your assets to work?

Arlene had always been very dependent on her husband. When he died, she despaired of being able to survive. But in talking with others, Arlene came to believe she could be a resourceful person. She determined to learn to drive a car and then find work outside her home. Within six months Arlene had a driver's license and a job. Now she could begin redirecting her emotions and energies. This is important, because a tragic loss often damages our self-esteem and results in a sense of lethargy and helplessness. Listing our personal assets and setting short-term goals will help us overcome those problems.

At some point we may need to do something good for ourselves to get back on track—especially if depression starts sinking in. A new suit or new hairdo, going out with a friend, taking the kids to the beach—these things can jar us out of the rut of self-pity.

All this also helps us get a hold on our own identity. Several months after losing her husband, Helen Raley decided to take a trip to the small Texas town where she had grown up. Helen drove past the familiar town square, the gin and cotton mill, and over the railroad tracks to the old farm. She met an old friend. They talked of places where they had played as children. Helen climbed the hill where Mama and Papa were buried and looked out over the familiar green valley, the sparkling river, and nodding trees. So much came back. She remembered all the love and dignity and hard work that had been part of her family.

Helen came to understand better who she was—and was able to go on and build a productive life. She realized that God still had plans for her.

As we regain a sense of our value in God's sight, we can better relate to the value of the person we have lost. They are gone, but their good works, their good qualities, live on after them. We can be thankful for that. We can begin to praise God for that. At this point we can begin to say with the psalmist: "Why are you in despair, O my soul? . . . Hope in God, for I shall again praise Him for the help of His presence." Psalm 42:5, NASB.

In writing about his own grief over the loss of his wife, C. S. Lewis wrote, "Praise is the mode of love which always has some element of joy in it. Praise in due order; of Him as the giver, of her as the gift. Don't we in praise somehow enjoy what we praise, however far we are from it?"

Praise keeps the loved one in perspective. It turns us from morbid recollections to cherished memories. The good qualities of a lost loved one can be a motivating force in our lives if we use them rightly. Some idolize the deceased and try to live according to the imagined wishes of the loved one. They, in effect, substitute the life of the departed for their own. This, in the end, is unhealthy. It becomes a trap. Remember that God has a plan for you, individually. His will is the only trustworthy guide for your life. What loved ones *can* do is to serve as examples that inspire.

Frank Deford was devastated by the death of his daughter, Alexandra. Cystic fibrosis had claimed her life at the age of eight. Several months after the funeral the question of adoption came up. Perhaps the Defords could adopt another girl. Chris, their son, thought it was a great idea. But Frank was reluctant. Giving some needy child a home was certainly a good thing, but Frank just couldn't think of bringing in some stranger to take Alexandra's place. It seemed terribly unfair. No one could ever replace her in their home.

But then one evening Frank's wife remarked, "You know, if we wanted to get a baby, we could probably never get one in the States. It would have to come from some far-away country." Yes, Frank understood that. Then his wife asked, "Do you remember Alexandra's prayer, the part she made up herself and said every night?" Yes, Frank remembered. His daughter had always prayed, "And God, please take care of our country, and bring some of the poor people to our country."

Tears came to Frank's eyes. Now he understood. Adopting another girl wouldn't replace Alexandra—it would answer her prayer. Within a few months the Defords had welcomed into their home a precious orphan girl from the Philippines. Now they could go on, rebuilding their lives. The idealism of a child had moved them to action. Frank later wrote, "We'll just have to start up again and go on from here. But thank you very much, Alexandra, because we do have a great deal to work with since you came our way."

What we have received from departed loved ones does give us "more to work with." It is tragic if we imprison ourselves in some morbid devotion to the deceased. That is a betrayal of the life they shared with us. How much better to build a fruitful life, inspired by their ideals.

Many people wonder how long it takes to recover from grief. When can we finally dry our tears? Well, counselors tell us that the period of mourning varies greatly with individuals. But we can be aware of one warning signal: one phase of grief dominating for more than several months.

Many of those who mourn go through periods of shock, anger, confusion, and depression. We work through our grief from one stage to another. But if, for example, we are still in shock four months after a tragedy, something is wrong. If depression goes on and on for a year, we may need professional help.

Nothing is really smooth in the process of grief. We will start and stop, experience peace—and then a sudden jab of bitter pain. But slowly, over time, we make progress. The ragged edge of memory begins to soften. The shrouded face of nature brightens; we begin to hear birds again and notice sunlight sparkling on the leaves. The gate to heaven, which seemed bolted shut, creaks open, and we are able to hear again Christ's invitation, "Come to Me, all who are weary and heavy laden." Matthew 11:28, NASB. Slowly we discover that He is indeed the "God of all comfort." 2 Corinthians 1:3.

And please let me assure you, God's comfort is not cheap. You invest your hopes and dreams, your very life in another precious life. You watch that person blossom and grow. And then suddenly, without explanation, that person is gone. You reach out to touch the loved one, but nothing is there. You beg, you plead, but there's no response.

Only in that terrible dark, in that aching emptiness, can we truly know the God of all comfort. Because only there can we find the fellowship of Christ's suffering. Yes, the Bible tells us that we can have fellowship, intimate fellowship, with Christ in His sufferings. Our time of grief can help us understand the depth of His love. It builds in us a deeper compassion and understanding.

Is there pain in grief? Yes. Darkness, moments of despair? Yes. But is it all meaningless and wasted? No! Not with the God of all comfort. Out of suffering, He fashions a new purpose. In our darkest hour, He draws us close. This God can show us the other side of mourning. You too can know this God of all comfort, this man acquainted with grief, whom to know is life eternal.

The Miracle of Hunza

Come with me on a once-in-a-lifetime journey to the rooftop of the world, the land of mountain giants, high in the Himalayas. We pass through the Karakorums, their peaks averaging more than 20,000 feet. Nine of them, standing shoulder to shoulder, lift their fingers more than 25,000 feet into a flawless sky. Having boarded a plane in Rawalpindi, in northeast Pakistan, we begin our descent into the ancient trading town of Gilgit—as far as we can fly.

This is a journey to Shangri-La. We're searching for the fountain of youth. Only 68 miles by jeep over the new Karakorum Highway separates us from the heart of Hunza, paradise of the Himalayas.

After a heart-stopping ride around sheer cliffs, we arrive at the valley of Hunza, just a few kilometers from the borders of China, Russia, and Afghanistan. The beauty of the valley takes our breath away. Emerald terraces on the mountainsides are bathed in sunlight. It is as if the Creator had hung baskets of living green between heaven and earth. The very air here is exhilarating.

The terraces, in reality, are the orchards and gardens of the Hunza people. In the absence of level land, they must carve out their gardens on nearly vertical slopes. Everywhere, it seems, the view is straight up. Especially magnificent Rakaposhi. The 25,500-foot peak is incredibly beautiful—and awesomely close. Michael Winn described Rakaposhi at dusk: "Standing three vertical miles higher than the valley, the mountain glowed like a jewel bathed in a soft white laser beam for several hours after the sun had set and the valley had become dark."

Michael commented, "Most of the peasants seemed to bear their poverty with a certain lightheartedness not found in the slums of Asian cities. It was as if life couldn't be too ugly if one lived in the lap of Mount Rakaposhi."

Looking down from the slopes of that towering peak to the valley floor, we see the palace of the king and queen—here known as the Mir and Rani—of Hunza. There too are homes far removed from the sophistication of New York, Paris, or London. There, cradled in the lap of Rakaposhi, are the people—hardy, tireless, seemingly ageless. They are the most fascinating part of this beautiful hideaway.

On a recent trip to this magnificent land, my family and I took time to admire again the skillfully landscaped terraces where men and women put in long hours cultivating—seemingly without fatigue—and have energy left for the evening.

We drank the refreshing water that comes down from nearby glaciers. The people call it "glacial milk" because of its milky appearance. This mineral-laden water is also used to irrigate the gardens and orchards.

The highlight of our trip to Hunza, of course, was visiting with the Mir and Rani. We were there as their guests and slept in guest rooms on the palace grounds. My wife, Nellie, and I, our three grandchildren, Shelli, Bradley, and Craig, with their mother, Judy, were royally entertained at their table. Ours was a people-to-people project to discover the secrets of their longevity. That's why the grandchildren were with us. They helped tremendously to make it a project long to be remembered.

The Mir and Rani are a delightful young couple—both of them only 34 years of age. We found them quiet, intelligent, and completely dedicated to helping their people in every possible way. It is easy to see why their subjects are so content. I'd like to share with you our interview with them as we sat in their beautiful reception room.

(GEV) Mir, tomorrow morning we're going to be taken into

the historic castle where your family has ruled for centuries. Could you tell us how long?

(MIR) My family has lived in Hunza and ruled this small state for about 960 years.

(GEV) Nine-hundred-sixty years? Nearly a thousand! And the same family?

(MIR) Yes. From father to son and from father to son.

(GEV) Remarkable! That must be a record.

(MIR) Yes, our family is one of the oldest families of the ruling families in Pakistan.

(GEV) You'd certainly be the one to answer this next question. That is about your roots, the origin of Hunza. I understand it dates back to the days of Alexander and his army passing through.

(MIR) Yes, after the fall of Alexander the Great, some of the Greek soldiers came and settled in this area. And the local population here, you know, are three main races—Iranians, Greeks, and Mongols. Our family is from Iran. The rest of the population are Greek descendants and Mongols.

(GEV) There's a little feature in that story that's interesting. Tradition has it that several Greek soldiers went AWOL or absconded from the army and came up the Hunza River when it was frozen. And by springtime, of course, no one could follow them—so difficult was the access. They were hidden here for years and finally established Hunza, about 2300 years ago. Is this part of the story true?

(Mir) Yes, I think so. Because at that time there were no roads, and it would be very difficult to reach this valley. So in the springtime it was much easier for them to come through the passes and settle in this area.

(Nellie) I would like to ask you, Rani, a little of your background. Would you tell us a little about how you became the Rani of Hunza?

(Rani) My husband and I met in the university. We were together there. We took a degree in political science. That is how we got married after the two families had agreed.

When my father-in-law died in 1976, my husband was asked by the people to come back. So we love to stay here and serve the people and do whatever we can for them.

(Nellie) I think that's wonderful. And the adjustment was not too hard on you?

(Rani) No, it wasn't. I should say, it wasn't hard for me.

(Nellie) Also, you had not even been to Hunza, had you, until you came here as the Rani?

(Rani) No, after I got married—that was the first time I came here. And I found everything beautiful.

(Nellie) Well, I can understand why. This is certainly one of the most beautiful spots on the face of the earth.

(GEV) Yes, and it's no secret why we're here. We're anxious to discover the reasons for the longevity that you've been famous for all these years.

(Mir) According to my thinking, there are a few reasons for this. First of all, we have very good food, which accounts a lot for the health of the people.

(Rani) It's a very simple diet. Unrefined.

(GEV) Don't you think that's the secret?

(Rani) I think that's the greatest secret.

(Mir) I think also because people have less worries. Because it is a settled area, and people are very friendly. And everyone in Hunza has a piece of land and a house. They are neither very rich nor very poor. They more or less belong to one class. And then you don't have to go for the income tax and property tax and all those things. We are away from these problems, so there are fewer worries. This also accounts a lot for the health of our people.

Anytime they need anything they can come to us for help. If they have any problem—it might be medical, it might be personal, or something else—they're most welcome. Therefore, we have a very friendly relationship with the population. They can come anytime they like. They can meet us, they can talk to us, and we're always here to help them. This is another reason the people live long.

(GEV) Is it true that there hasn't been a crime reported here for many years?

(Mir) Well, this is not an area of high crime. We don't have any murders, rapes, kidnappings, and all that. We have small problems—dispute problems, land problems—which we settle ourselves according to the Islamic law. We have not had murders for years and years. We are very lucky.

(GEV) We were talking the other day, Rani, about our Seventh-day Adventist hospital in Karachi and how the royal family through the years has traveled there for certain emergencies. And we thought about the hospital situation in the United States and how the cost of medical services has grown astronomically. Then you made an interesting statement. Would you mind repeating it?

(Rani) Well, I just said that in Hunza we don't have any hospitals.

(GEV) You don't need them?

(Rani) We don't need them because nature is very kind to the people, and we don't have any diseases such as cancer and things like that. I think that from the very beginning the people developed an immunity from these diseases. They are so close to nature over here, and nature is really kind to them.

(GEV) I notice you say that nature is very kind. We need to cooperate with nature, too, don't you think? And evidently you people have been cooperating.

(Rani) We are in such a remote area. We have fresh air and fresh water, and these other things account for the longevity of the Hunza people and for their good health. Cancer is such a common disease these days all over the world. But thank God we don't have it.

(GEV) And heart trouble? How about heart trouble?

(Rani) We have not heard of a single heart patient over here.

(GEV) There's no oil in your Hunza bread. I believe you don't use oil in cooking like we use it.

(Rani) No, we don't use it.

(GEV) We understand this is the culprit—one of the causes of heart disease.

(Rani) Yes, you can say so. Of course, the life of the people is very hard, you know. They work very hard and exercise hard, you see. And then they eat very simply and have a very good diet, which is what they have been doing for centuries.

(GEV) You've demonstrated it right here at your table. Absolutely delectable. Listen, folks, may the dear God bless you in your heavy responsibilities, both of you. And thank you so much for spending these moments with us.

It becomes apparent, as we look at the Hunza lifestyle more closely, that diet is one of the key factors which contributes to their longer life. Now some may say, "I don't think I could take it. It would be too rigid, too restricted." But let me assure you that the food in Hunza is good and wholesome.

Unfortunately, any suggestion of a more healthful diet conjures up all sorts of unpleasant ideas. We seem to think that everything that is good for us must surely taste terrible. Vegetables! And whole grains! Maybe dying young wouldn't be so bad!

Is it possible that we have so accustomed ourselves to fast food and highly spiced dishes, so stimulated ourselves with coffee and cocktails, and made of ourselves such sugar addicts that we have missed the real luxuries? Have we covered our vegetables with vinegar and mustard and catsup and garlic until we can't even savor the delectable flavor of the vegetables themselves? How can we know what an avocado really tastes like if we smother it with dressing? Just a little salt would bring out its natural, delicious flavor.

You may have eaten Harvard beets, or pickled beets. But do you know how very tasty small hot buttered beets can be?

Try preparing vegetables more simply, not cooking them so long, and give them a chance. Try adding just a little butter or margarine, or a little milk or cream, or maybe a cream sauce—and see what you've been missing!

Healthful eating doesn't have to be a lot of dos and don'ts. Listen to what the prophet Isaiah said: "Wherefore do ye spend money for that which is not bread? and your labour for that which satisfieth not? hearken diligently unto me, and eat ye that which is good." Isaiah 55:2.

Eating that which is good. That's real healthful living. That's the winning diet! Evidently God thought fruits and vegetables and grains and nuts were good. Listen to what He provided for our first parents: "And God said, Behold, I have given you every herb bearing seed, which is upon the face of all the earth, and every tree, in the which is the fruit of a tree yielding seed; to you it shall be for meat." Genesis 1:29. Simply stated, that's fruits, grains, and nuts. Vegetables were added later.

Could it be that the closer we get to the original Eden diet, the better off we will be? After all, the God who created us ought to know best what to put into the bodies He made.

Although the Hunza people do eat some meat, especially in winter when fresh foods are not available, their diet is amazingly similar to the diet in Eden. Is it any wonder they live longer?

Seventh-day Adventists, who recommend the elimination of meat from the diet, have come still closer to the original plan. And what has happened? Since they don't smoke, they have almost no lung cancer. And even with all the stresses of civilization, they live an average of six to seven years longer than their neighbors.

According to a National Academy of Sciences survey of cancer and nutrition studies, a diet low in fat, including whole grain cereal products, and emphasizing the importance of fruits and vegetables—especially vegetables that contain vitamin A—might be the best way to reduce your risk of cancer.

Dr. T. Colin Campbell of Cornell University says, "Diet, which appears to be associated with most cancers, may be the single most important risk factor for cancer." This distinguished nutritionist also states that a poor diet can increase cancer risk tenfold.

Hard to eat healthfully? Hard to be vegetarian? It certainly becomes easier when we discover the facts about diet, disease, and health.

No trip to Hunza would be complete without visiting the homes of the people. In order to get a closer look at their healthful lifestyle, we stopped by the warm and friendly home of Haji Sahib. Haji is 75 years old. But you would never know it by his daily routine.

(GEV) Haji, how many children to you have?

(Haji) I have three sons and four daughters.

(GEV) Tell me, what has been your work through the years? Have you been a farmer?

(Haji) Yes, I am a farmer.

(GEV) Near your home here? Or do you have to go a distance?

(Haji) No, my fields are only one mile from my house.

(GEV) Do you walk it?

(Haji) Yes, I walk it.

(GEV) Good exercise. That's been good for you, hasn't it?

(Haji) I go to my fields. I seed my fields. And when I was young I plowed my fields, and I still plow.

(GEV) What do you grow?

(Haji) Wheat, barley, maize, buckwheat.

(GEV) Do you have any orchards with apricots?

(Haji) Yes, the garden is near my home.

(GEV) Your various fruit trees are there?

(Haji) I have apricots in my garden and some apples, but I do not have grapes.

(GEV) We tasted some of Hunza's grapes the other day. They were delicious.

While visiting with the Haji family, Nellie was able to talk with the mother, Mrs. Haji, about her daily life.

(Nellie) It's so nice of you to let us come to your home, Mrs. Haji.

(Mrs. Haji) You are most welcome. I love my guests so much.

(Nellie) One thing I have been very impressed with is how warm and friendly the Hunza people are.

(Mrs. Haji) We enjoy having our guests, especially those who are from out of the country.

(Nellie) Thank you. You've raised such a large family, and I know you have to spend a lot of time in the home. But do you spend quite a bit of time in the fields as well?

(Mrs. Haji) I have to go to the fields to work. I work there for three hours and cultivate many things like wheat, barley, and buckwheat. Then I come home to do the rest of my work, making things in the house—like spinning and embroidery.

(Nellie) You make your own cloth then?

(Mrs. Haji) I've never been to the tailor. And I make all the things for my husband and for my children.

Plainly, the people of Hunza lead active, vigorous lives. Their regular exercise is unquestionably another of the big factors in their longevity and physical fitness. That became especially apparent as we watched old and young compete in an exciting game of polo. This is actually the land where polo originated, and many here enjoy the sport.

These people seem remarkably free from fatigue. The men can walk the sixty-eight miles from Gilgit and go right out to the fields and work as if they had just had a nap. Hunza men once carried a piano all the way from Gilgit. And the women work long hours in the fields and then do all their chores at home—seemingly without fatigue. One more thing, there is no overweight problem in Hunza. During our stay in that country, I didn't see one single obese citizen.

The reasons why the Hunza people don't die young have become clearer. Good diet. Exercise. Fresh air. Fresh water. And, of course, they get plenty of sleep at night.

We might also mention sunlight. It too must be a major factor. The Hunza people are exceptionally happy. Their little paradise is bathed in sunlight. But there are people on the other side of Mount Rakaposhi who are kept in shade much of the time. And those people, though they have a similarly healthful lifestyle, are more irritable and quarrelsome. I'm told they are so irritable that mountain climbers will not hire them as porters.

It would be a mistake to emphasize any one factor in the Hunza lifestyle to the exclusion of the others. It would especially be a mistake to underestimate the importance of the religious life in Hunza—their trust in a divine being.

I discussed this aspect of Hunza culture with Peter Wylie, the senior master of the distinguished Wellington School in England. He has through the years made an intensive study of Islam, the official religion of Hunza, and its many sects. He too was a guest of the Mir and Rani when we were there.

(GEV) Peter, tell us a little about Islam. How many different sects are there?

(Wylie) There are three main sects, if one likens them to the Protestant or Catholic church denominations. There are the Shiites, who are equivalent to the Catholics. There are the Sunnites—that is the Protestant group, and then there's a third sect, the Ismailis, which I am particularly interested in, who owe their allegiance to the Aga Khan, and are sort of midway between the two.

(GEV) What part then does the Mir play in the spiritual leadership of the people?

(Wylie) Well, George, the Mir is absolutely fascinating, and so is his office. His ancestral castle goes back 900 years. There are two branches of Ismailiism. The branch in Hunza owes its origin to a mystic, traveler, poet, and deep thinker who lived in Afghanistan. He sent his messengers across these magnificent mountains and converted these people here. His message was the message of peace, of reconciliation. No warfare.

A lot of Islam involves the sword. But with the Ismailis, there was cooperation, peace, and love for your neighbor. And it's been in this particular valley for 900 years, unbroken, unceasing. This message has been lived out, not just preached, but lived in the lives of the Hunzakuts here.

(GEV) That's been very helpful, Peter. You as a Britisher and practicing Anglican, and I as a Protestant from the United States, can have fellowship with these people because we both worship the same God. Allah is simply another name, of course, for God. Naturally, you and I believe that there is a greater revelation in Jesus Christ, who makes God real and brings salvation to us personally, but we can have some genuine fellowship, and that's good.

Peter, does the faith we've been describing here assist in stabilizing the home?

(Wylie) Oh yes, very much. The whole thing is home-based, family-based, community-based.

I do believe that the faith of the Hunza people, with its emphasis on the peace and love of God, also contributes to their amazing health. They live remarkably worry-free, stress-free lives. Lifting our sights, lifting our confidence above every earthly thing to the great God who created us and our world does wonders for our health and peace of mind.

After looking closely at the "miracle of Hunza" and examining their lifestyle, I'm not so sure that Hunza longevity is such a miracle after all. A miracle is something in which the laws of nature are overruled—something contrary to the way things usually happen. If a loaded gun does not fire when the trigger is pulled, and a life is spared, that's a miracle. If a man loses an eye in an accident, leaving him with an empty socket, and suddenly he has a new eye, that's a miracle. Nature simply doesn't work that way.

But if a family is brought up in natural surroundings, with fresh, unpolluted air, pure water, a simple, appetizing diet, plenty of sunshine, plenty of sleep, an abundance of exercise and a minimum of worry—is it a miracle if that family has excellent health? Isn't it just what you would expect under the circumstances?

How often have you heard commercials assuring you that if you overeat, just take Brand X and everything will be OK? I haven't heard too many telling us *not* to overeat so we won't need Brand X. Today's philosophy is "Eat as you please. Live as you please. Just take Brand X."

But there comes a time when Brand X doesn't work anymore. Overeating, inactivity, and other health-destroying habits result in serious illness. It's a simple matter of cause and effect. Paul the apostle said, "Be not deceived; God is not mocked: for whatsoever a man soweth, that shall he also reap." Galatians 6:7. Cause and effect, you see. It works with mathematical precision.

Jesus healed many people. But He didn't heal promiscuously. He saw no point in healing a man who would return immediately to the lifestyle that would make him ill again. Jesus never separated His healing from His teaching. He said to one man He had healed, "Behold, thou art made whole: sin no more, lest a worse thing come unto thee." John 5:14.

Sometimes we're just a little dull, a little slow to get the message. A woman was injured once when a spark from a lighted match flew into her eye. She went to her eye doctor. He thought this might be a good time to encourage her to stop smoking. So he said, "Maybe that match was trying to tell you something."

"I think so," she replied. "I'm going to go right out and get a lighter."

The price of good health is not a new lighter; it's a change in lifestyle. And the real miracle of Hunza may be that 55,000 people are willing, even content, to follow a lifestyle that makes them the envy of the world. Can the same be said of you and me?

A pictorial review
of It Is Written's
memorable people-to-people
mission to Hunza

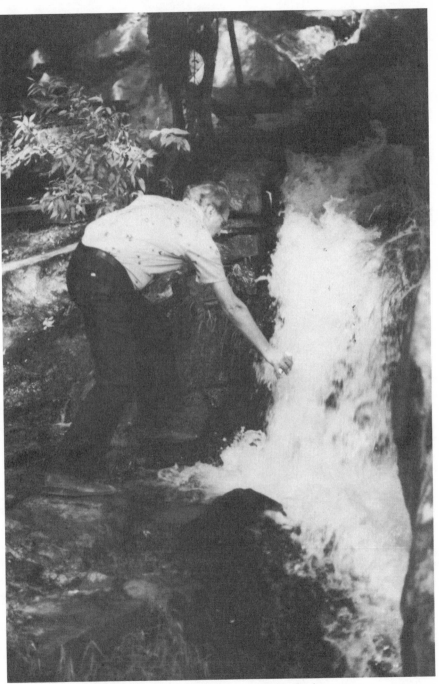

George Vandeman samples sparkling glacier water.

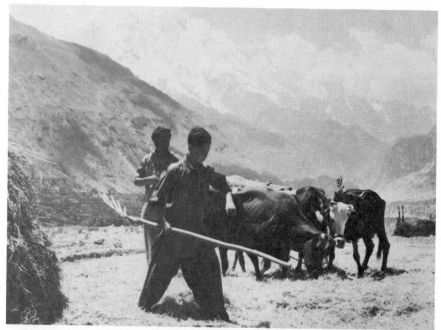

Towering mountains provide a backdrop for work.

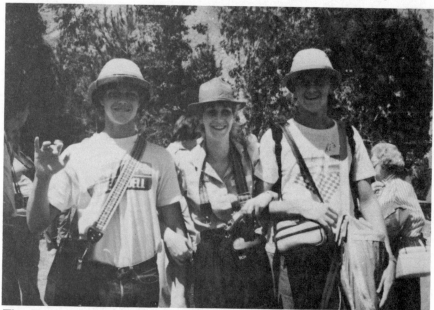

The Vandeman grandchildren, Craig, Shellie, and Brad, arrive in Hunza
with the camera crew to act their part in a people-to-people mission.

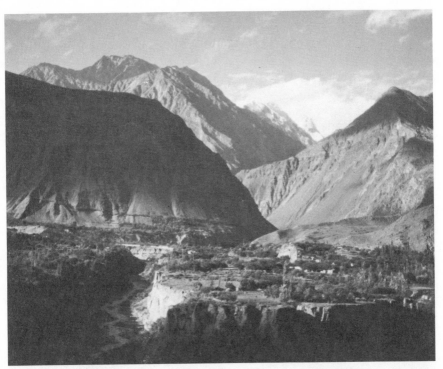

Terraces seem suspended between earth and sky.

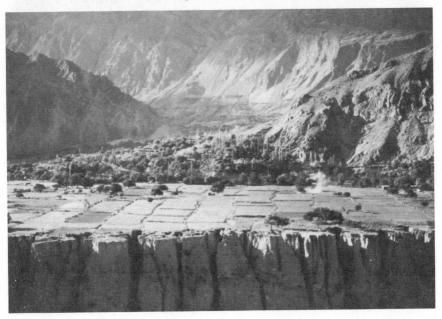

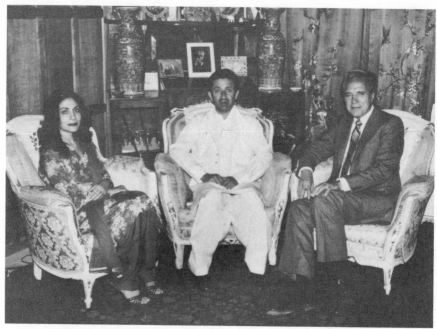
George Vandeman visiting the Mir and Rani of Hunza.

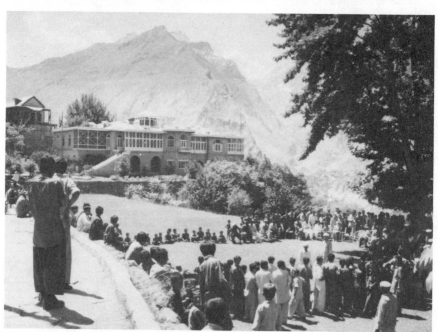
Royal palace in Hunza.

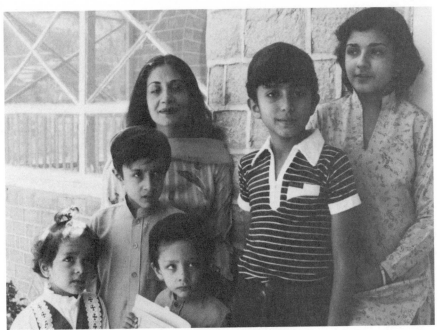

The Rani and her family.

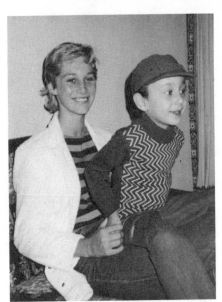

Shellie and the Mir's eldest child.

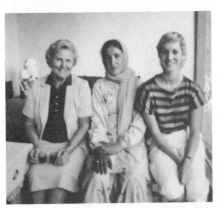

Nellie Vandeman and Shellie visit
with the Hajis' daughter.

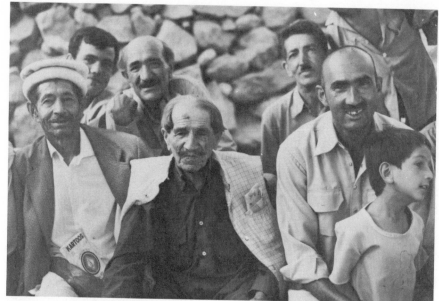

Hunzakuts with a 120-year-old citizen.

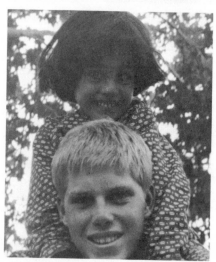

Craig playing with a Hunza child.

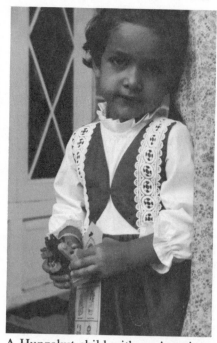

A Hunzakut child with an American
gift toy in her hand.

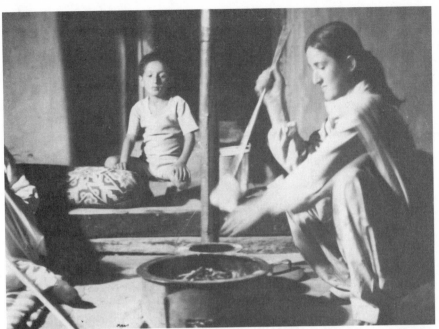

Hunzakut woman preparing to bake bread.

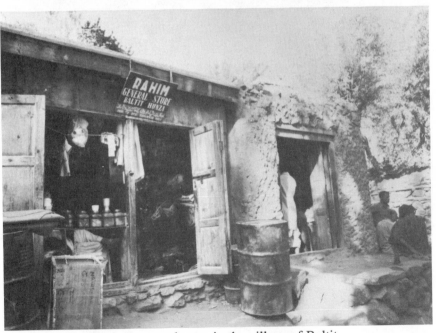

Typical general store in the village of Baltit.

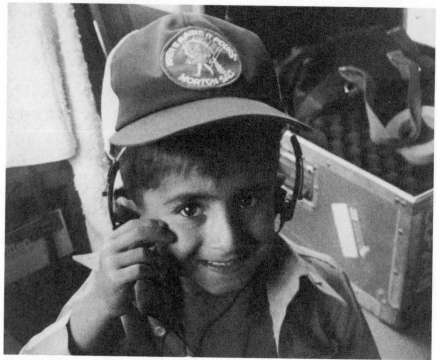

This little fellow had no shoes. Brad bought him a pair, and he didn't leave Brad's side till departure day.